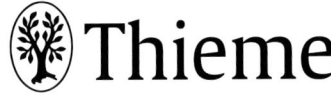

Nonsurgical Therapies for the Gut and Abdominal Cavity

Edited by

Jeffrey C. Brandon, M.D.
Vice Chairman
Department of Radiology
University of South Alabama
Mobile, AL

Steven K. Teplick, M.D.
Chairman
Department of Radiology
University of South Alabama
Mobile, AL

2001
Thieme
New York · Stuttgart

SOUTH UNIVERSITY
709 MALL BLVD.
SAVANNAH, GA 31406

Thieme New York
333 Seventh Avenue
New York, NY 10001

Editor: Kathleen P. Lyons
Editorial Assistant: Diane Sardini
Director, Production & Manufacturing: Anne Vinnicombe
Production Editor: Felicity Edge
Marketing Director: Phyllis Gold
Sales Manager: Ross Lumpkin
Chief Financial Officer: Peter van Woerden
President: Brian D. Scanlan
Cover Designer: Kevin Kall
Compositor: The PRD Group
Printer: The Sheridan Press

Library of Congress Cataloging-in-Publication Data

Brandon, Jeffrey C.
  Nonsurgical therapies for the gut and abdominal cavity / Jeffrey C. Brandon, Steven K. Teplick.
     p. ; cm.
  Includes bibliographical references and index.
  ISBN 0-86577-997-X (hard cover : alk. paper)
    1. Gastrointestinal system—Diseases—Diagnosis. 2. Gastrointestinal system—Imaging.
  3. Interventional radiology. 4. Abdomen—Radiography. 5.
  Abdomen—Diseases—Diagnosis. I. Teplick, Steven K. II. Title.
    [DNLM: 1. Gastrointestinal Diseases—therapy. 2. Radiography,
  Interventional—methods. WI 140 B819n 2001]
  RC804.D52 B73 2001
  616.3'3075—dc21   2001027189

Copyright © 2001 by Thieme Medical Publishers, Inc. This book, including all parts thereof, is legally protected by copyright. Any use, exploitation or commercialization outside the narrow limits set by copyright legislation, without the publisher's consent, is illegal and liable to prosecution. This applies in particular to photostat reproduction, copying, mimeographing or duplication of any kind, translating, preparation of microfilms, and electronic data processing and storage.

Important note: Medical knowledge is ever-changing. As new research and clinical experience broaden our knowledge, changes in treatment and drug therapy may be required. The authors and editors of the material herein have consulted sources believed to be reliable in their efforts to provide information that is complete and in accord with the standards accepted at the time of publication. However, in view of the possibility of human error by the authors, editors, or publisher of the work herein, or changes in medical knowledge, neither the authors, editors, publisher, nor any other party who has been involved in the preparation of this work, warrants that the information contained herein is in every respect accurate or complete, and they are not responsible for any errors or omissions or for the results obtained from use of such information. Readers are encouraged to confirm the information contained herein with other sources. For example, readers are advised to check the product information sheet included in the package of each drug they plan to administer to be certain that the information contained in this publication is accurate and that changes have not been made in the recommended dose or in the contraindications for administration. This recommendation is of particular importance in connection with new or infrequently used drugs.

Some of the product names, patents, and registered designs referred to in this book are in fact registered trademarks or proprietary names even though specific reference to this fact is not always made in the text. Therefore, the appearance of a name without designation as proprietary is not to be construed as a representation by the publisher that it is in the public domain.

Printed in the United States of America

5 4 3 2 1

TNY ISBN 1-86577-997-X
GTV ISBN WN 21466

Contents

Contributors vii

Preface ix

Acknowledgment xi

1. Gastrointestinal Bleeding: A Multidisciplinary Approach 1
   Kristine J. Kreuger, Lane S. Kannegieter, and Christine Evankovich

2. Gastrointestinal Stenting: Indications and Techniques 35
   Mark G. Cowling and Andreas Adam

3. Percutaneous Gastrostomy, Gastroenterostomy,
   and Jejunostomy 51
   David D. Kidney and Larry-Stuart Deutsch

4. Percutaneous Colostomy 77
   Lorenzo Carson and Elvira Lang

5. Peritoneal/Retroperitoneal Anatomy: Relevance to
   Performance of Interventional Procedures 95
   John P. McGahan, R. Brooke Jeffrey, Jr., and Michael J. Lane

   Index 117

Contributors

Andreas Adam, F.R.C.P., F.R.C.R.
Professor of Interventional Radiology
Department of Interventional Radiology
St. Thomas' Hospital
London, UK

Lorenzo Carson, M.D.
Radiology Associates of Albany
Albany, GA

Mark G. Cowling, M.R.C.P., F.R.C.R.
Consultant Radiologist
Department of Radiology
St. Mary's Hospital
London, UK

Larry-Stuart Deutsch, M.D., C.M., F.R.C.P.C.
Professor and Chief of Service
Vascular and Interventional Radiology
University of Nebraska
Omaha, NE

Christine Evankovich, M.D.
Assistant Professor
Department of Surgery
University of South Alabama Medical Center
Mobile, AL

R. Brooke Jeffrey, Jr., M.D.
Professor
Department of Radiology
Stanford University Medical Center
Stanford, CA

Lane Kannegieter, M.D.
Associate Professor
Department of Radiology
University of South Alabama Medical Center
Mobile, AL

David D. Kidney, M.B., M.R.C.P.I., F.E.R., F.R.C.R., M.Sc.
Associate Professor of Radiology
Department of Radiological Sciences
University of California
Irvine Medical Center
Orange, CA

Kristine Krueger, M.D.
Associate Professor of Medicine
Department of Gastroenterology/Internal Medicine
University of Louisville
Louisville, KY

Michael J. Lane, M.D.
Section Chief
Department of Radiology
Brooke Army Medical Center
Fort Sam Houston, TX

Elvira V. Lang, M.D.
Associate Professor of Radiology and Medicine
Department of Radiology
Harvard School of Medicine
Beth Israel Deaconess Hospital
Boston, MA

John P. McGahan, M.D.
Professor
Director of Abdominal Imaging and Ultrasound
Department of Radiology
University of California Davis Medical Center
Sacramento, CA

Preface

The purpose of this book is to familiarize readers with established or emerging interventional techniques used in the esophagus, stomach, and intestines. The book concludes with descriptions of procedures relevant to the peritoneal cavity because of its intimate relationship to the intra-abdominal portion of these organs. Not infrequently, the percutaneous or transluminal methods described in this text have replaced more traditional surgical approaches. However, the complexity of certain gastrointestinal disorders frequently demands a multidisciplinary focus to best serve the patient. Management of gastrointestinal bleeding is such an example. The authors of the first chapter—a gastroenterologist, a radiologist, and a surgeon—combine their experiences to offer insight into this challenging problem. Subsequent chapters cover the remarkable progress radiologists have made intervening in the digestive tube from the hypopharynx to the colon, and we are fortunate to have many of those responsible for these advances as contributing authors. The figures were chosen to provide enough detail to radiologists interested in attempting those procedures, and the text should convey the judgment and technical insight necessary to perform them successfully. We are indebted to the authors for investing the time and effort to help compile this information. Our hope is that radiologists will find the material in this book to be useful in their clinical practice and of benefit to their patients.

Jeffrey C. Brandon, M.D.
Steven K. Teplick, M.D.

Acknowledgment

The authors thank Deborah Hoang for her assistance in the preparation of the manuscript.

Chapter 1

Gastrointestinal Bleeding: A Multidisciplinary Approach

Kristine J. Krueger
Lane S. Kannegieter
Christine Evankovich

Gastrointestinal (GI) hemorrhage results in 250,000 to 300,000 U.S. hospital admissions each year, with bleeding due to peptic ulceration accounting for a significant number of these admissions.[1,2] The epidemiologic aspect of GI bleeding is complex and dynamic:[3-5] gastric ulcer rates have increased over the past several decades in part due to the common use of nonsteroidal anti-inflammatory drugs (NSAIDs).[6-8] Furthermore, *Helicobacter pylori* infection rates also increase with age. Although not yet fully understood, the importance of *H. pylori* in ulcer pathogenesis is now widely recognized.[9] Lastly, vascular anomalies, such as angiodysplasias, are recognized more often as a source of upper, small intestinal, and lower GI bleeding.[10] These are often multiple and bleed intermittently, posing added challenges to their diagnosis and management.

Despite improved medical and surgical care, the overall 6 to 7% mortality for GI hemorrhage has not improved in more than two decades, possibly because of the comorbidity of our increasingly elderly population.[1,5] Limitations in medical therapy for actively bleeding ulcers helped pave the road for advancements in fiberoptic technology such that by the early 1980s it was routine practice to perform early endoscopy in bleeding patients.[11,12] Over the last decade and a half, endoscopic therapeutic applications for patients with active bleeding or visible vessels at endoscopy (including injection therapy, laser, and thermal coagulation) have resulted in reduced hopital stays, decreased transfusion requirements, significantly reduced bleeding and rebleeding, and decreased need for emergency surgery.[11] Meta-analysis of endoscopic hemostatic therapies for nonvariceal upper GI hemorrhage also confirms a significant reduction in mortality.[13] Surgical laparoscopists are now able to apply minimally invasive surgery for the treatment of small bowel and gastric lesions that are not amenable to endoscopic methods.[14,15] The appropriate use of interventional radiologic techniques has also complemented the diagnosis and definitive management of many bleeding GI lesions.[16-19]

In many instances, choosing a gastroenterologic, surgical, or radiologic approach to GI bleeding is determined by local expertise and experience. The clinical impact of managed care and the adoption of practice guidelines may also be influential. More than ever before, clinical gatekeepers must be familiar with the specific utility and the predictive value of diagnostic tests and therapeutic procedures in their bleeding patients. Finally, more studies comparing costs, follow-up care, and long-term outcome are needed to clarify which techniques or therapies are most appropriate for the individual patient.

Upper Gastointestinal Bleeding

Medical Resuscitation

Because an estimated 70 to 80% of GI bleeding stops spontaneously, the clinician's primary objective is to prevent damage to vital organs from hypoperfusion.[20] Bleeding from upper GI sources may be obvious when the patient presents with hematemesis, or occult in cases of severe iron deficiency anemia and Hemoccult-positive stool. Historical clues, including ulcer-type pain, use of NSAIDs, or underlying renal disease (risk for angiodysplasias) or liver disease (risk for portal hypertension), may be helpful. The presence of orthostatic hypotension indicates about 20% blood volume loss, whereas resting tachycardia, shock, azotemia, or lactic acidosis indicates major blood loss and need for intensive care.[21] The placement of a nasogastric (NG) tube can be helpful and predictive of outcome. Aspirating "coffee ground" material may help establish the upper GI tract as the source of bleeding. Obtaining fresh persistently red blood that does not "clear" with continued lavage is particularly ominous because the mortality increases to as high as 50% in such patients.[22,23] Caution is advised not to overinterpret a negative NG aspirate because the tube may be malpositioned in the esophagus or proximal stomach and therefore not representative of more distal contents. Aspiration of clear greenish bile–colored fluid indicates an adequate sample in a nonacutely bleeding patient but does not predict the chance of rebleeding. There is a generally recognized higher mortality from upper GI hemorrhage in elderly patients due to comorbidity and a higher likelihood of there being deeper ulcers in the gastric body.[24] Although controversial, there is no consensus on whether NSAID use as a cause of bleeding is associated with higher mortality compared with other causes of bleeding peptic ulcer.[25]

Effective resuscitative measures include the prompt establishment of intravenous access and administration of fluids and blood products. The formerly routine administration of fresh frozen plasma as well as packed red blood cells for patients with ongoing hemorrhage is outdated. However, patients with known specific factor deficiencies, cirrhotic patients,[26] and anticoagulated patients[27] may require plasma or specific replacement factors. Patients with altered mental status or who repeatedly vomit blood are at high risk for aspiration. Therefore, elective endotracheal intubation should be considered in these patients if urgent endoscopy is necessary for bleeding control.[28] Administration of the fluoroquinolone antibiotic norfloxacin in cirrhotic patients with acute bleeding has been shown to reduce infectious complications.[29] Pharmacologic treatment for the control of bleeding should be begun as early as possible, when indicated.

While resuscitating, clinicians should consult endoscopists, surgeons, and interventional radiologists for their collaborative input and subsequent management. About 20% of patients with upper GI hemorrhage will have continuous or intermittent bleeding. These are the patients with the highest overall mortality, and shock at presentation is the best clinical predictor of recurrent hemorrhage.[30]

Pharmacologic Control of Bleeding

Control of Acute Bleeding

Formerly, intravenous pitressin with or without nitroglycerin was used to control hemorrhage from esophageal and gastric varices. Pitressin causes splanchnic arteriolar constriction, resulting in 20 to 30% decreased portal and azygous venous pressure.[31] Nitroglycerin decreases splanchnic blood flow via venodilatation; its recommended use with pitressin is to combat the systemic side effects of coronary, renal, and mesenteric artery constriction, increased peripheral vascular resistance, and potential for ischemia.[32] Popular in the last decade, intravenous octreotide, a synthetic somatostatin analogue, has been proven effective and safe. Its mechanism of action, though not completely understood, includes directly increasing the pressure of the lower esophageal sphincter (tamponade effect) and reducing blood flow to the adjacent vasculature. Systemic effects include lowering of splanchnic pressure without increase in peripheral vascular resistance. Studies of octreotide alone and as an adjunct to sclerotherapy or band ligation of varices reveal its clinical usefulness in acutely controlling portal hypertensive bleeding.[33,34] A recent meta-analysis of the use of octreotide or somatostatin in hospitalized patients with endoscopically proven non-variceal-related upper GI hemorrhage found that treated patients were significantly less likely to rebleed or require surgery.[35]

Prevention of Portal Hypertensive Bleeding

Prophylactic therapy for the prevention of recurrent hemorrhage associated with portal hypertension cannot be overemphasized. Patients with esophageal and gastric varices or portal hypertensive gastropathy should be maintained on a noncardioselective β-blocker titrated to reduce the resting heart rate by 25%, which causes about a 25 to 30% reduction in portal pressure. Propranolol reduces the incidence of initial bleeding,[36] increases the time between bleeding episodes,[37] and is superior to sclerotherapy for the prevention of first bleeding.[38] It reduces heart rate and renal blood flow as well as portal pressure but is metabolized in the liver, so that metabolism may be erratic in cirrhotic patients. Common side effects include fatigue, sleep disturbances, and changes in libido, all limiting medical compliance. Nadolol, another noncardioselective β-blocker, also prevents first episodes of bleeding.[39,40] Because this drug does not affect renal blood flow and is not metabolized by the liver, it may emerge as the preferred β-blocker for chronic pharmacologic reduction of portal pressure. Many clinicians add nitrates to β-blocker therapy for added portal pressure reduction, or as single therapy for patients who are intolerant of β-blockers.[41] Experimentally, nitrates reduce mesenteric blood flow by venodilatation, resulting in a baroreceptor–mediated compensatory arterial vasoconstriction.[42] Nitrates may also reduce portal pressure by relaxation of the presinusoidal and septal myofibroblasts in the liver, resulting in decreased resistance to portal flow.[43,44] Hemodynamic studies of cirrhotic patients have demonstrated decreases in mean arterial pressure and in the hepatic vein pressure gradient with organic nitrates.[45–47] A study comparing β-blocker plus nitrates with nitrates alone revealed a greater reduction in the hepatic vein pressure gradient with combination therapy.[48] Whether the observed greater hemodynamic effect reduces the rate of rebleeding awaits the results of randomized clinical trials. Clonidine, a centrally acting α_2 agonist, has been shown to decrease portal pressure by decreasing postsinusoidal resistance and constricting the splanchnic circulation.[49] Controlled trials have not been performed comparing the efficacy of clonidine over β-blockers or nitrates. In a recent small randomized study of patients with biopsy-proven cirrhosis and variceal hemorrhage, the group receiving twice-daily subcutaneous injections of octreotide plus routine sclerotherapy had decreased mortality, decreased rebleeding, lower hepatic venous pressure, and overall improved hepatic function compared with the group that received sclerotherapy alone.[50]

Acid-Suppressive Therapy

Chronic acid suppression for maintaining remission of upper GI bleeding is indicated for erosive esophagitis or esophageal ulcers. Proton pump inhibitors are clinically and economically superior to H_2 receptor antagonists for acute and chronic healing of erosive esophagitis.[51] Proton pump inhibitors are superior to all other agents in reducing recurrent bleeding and ulceration associated with NSAID-induced gastric or duodenal ulcers.[52] They are recommended for any patient with a history of bleeding from NSAID-associated ulceration who continues to use these medications. Chronic acid suppression is recommended for patients with non-NSAID-associated bleeding who are not infected with *H. pylori*. In this group, representing less than 10% of ulcer patients, hypersecretory conditions should be excluded. Critically ill patients requiring mechanical ventilation have an increased risk of stress gastritis and should be treated prophylactically with acid-suppressive medicines.[53]

Helicobacter Pylori *Eradication*

At least 90% of non-NSAID-induced peptic ulcers are associated with *H. pylori* infection. Successful eradication of this organism results in significantly reduced rates of both recurrent ulceration[9,54] and recurrent bleeding.[55-57] Repeat upper endoscopy with biopsy or urease breath testing is justified in patients with prior *H. pylori*-induced bleeding ulcers to ensure eradication.[58] In 1992, a Consensus Development Conference of the National Institutes of Health recommended that all patients with ulcers who are infected with *H. pylori* receive antimicrobial therapy.[59] It will likely take decades before the impact of this recommendation is realized; it is predicted that the cost of *H. pylori* eradication will compare favorably with that of chronic acid suppression or surgery.

Endoluminal Management

Diagnostic Endoscopy

Traditionally, the term "upper GI bleeding" refers to bleeding mucosal lesions proximal to the ligament of Treitz. In most instances, standard upper endoscopic procedures expose very little of the hypopharyngeal mucosa, distal duodenum, or proximal jejunum. A carefully obtained bleeding history should allow the endoscopist to select the appropriate equipment, with an expected endoscopic diagnostic yield of 90 to 95%. Occasionally, retained blood clots obscure the bleeding site. Prior evacuation of the stomach with a large-bore Ewald or Edlich tube is often helpful. Patients can also be turned from the standard left lateral position to shift retained blood clots to more gravity-dependent areas. Lesions likely to be missed under fundic clots include Mallory-Weiss tears, gastric varices, Dieulafoy's lesion (a type of arteriovenous malformation), and malignancies. Peptic ulcer disease predictably causes ulcerations in the duodenal bulb, the immediate postbulbar region, the gastric antrum, and the lesser curvature of the gastric body. Even when the stomach is full of retained fluid and clots, these areas can usually be thoroughly examined. Nodular antral mucosa with patchy erythema may clue the endoscopist to the possibility of *H. pylori* infection, and a biopsy can be obtained at endoscopy for the presence of urease.[60] Esophageal varices are usually readily apparent; stigmata of recent bleeding include cherry-red spots and red whale markings. Gastric varices are often confused with prominent rugal folds, making their distinction less definite during endoscopy. About 50% of upper GI bleeding is due to peptic ulcer, and about 15% is from esophageal or gastric varices, with esophagitis, erosive duodenitis, Mallory-Weiss tears, portal hypertensive gastropathy, and vascular anomalies accounting for most of the remainder.[1,10,61,62] More obscure causes, such as Dieulafoy's lesion, watermelon stomach, duodenal varices, and pancreaticobiliary sources account for less than 2% of cases.[63-67]

When standard upper endoscopy fails to identify a bleeding site despite a history suggestive of upper GI bleeding, another endoscopy can be performed with a longer instrument. Adult or pediatric colonoscopes can usually be inserted to or just beyond the ligament of Treitz; small bowel push enteroscopes with or without an overtube can reach up to 1 m beyond the ligament of Treitz.[68,69] When the distal jejunum or proximal ileum warrants visualization, the sonde (pull) enteroscope may be useful. This instrument is 3 m long and 5 mm in diameter, allowing for transnasal (or transoral) passage. The entire small bowel can be traversed in as little as 4 to 6 hours. An estimated 50 to 75% of small intestinal mucosa is surveyed during the viewing (pulling back) portion of the examination.[70,71] Unlike all of the other modern endoscopes, therapeutic capabilities with the sonde have not been developed. The instrument tip can be deflected, and a balloon can be inflated to slow down the removal so that plain film x-rays or video can be obtained for future reference. Small bowel push enteroscopes, including the sonde, can be used in conjunction with laparotomy or laparoscopy for localization of bleeding sites prior to planned surgical interventions.[70] The diagnostic yield using these enteroscopes when standard endoscopy is unrevealing is 30 to 40%, and the main bleeding lesions encountered are vascular anomalies. Jejunal or ileal ulcers, bleeding diverticulae, and neoplasias are rarely found.[70,71]

Endoscopic Findings and Interventions Predict Outcomes

The endoscopic appearance of bleeding lesions is predictive of rebleeding rates, morbidity, mortality, and need for emergency surgery.[72–80] Because ulcers with a yellow–white "clean" base have a less than 5% risk of rebleeding, patients with clean-based ulcers may be discharged safely after medical stabilization and treatment. Ulcers with flat red or black spots either within them or along their edges have a less than 10% incidence of rebleeding (Fig. 1–1). An adherent clot has a rebleeding potential of about 25% because the clot may overlie a flat lesion or a protruding vessel (Fig. 1–2). Controversy exists as to whether it is advisable to dislodge a clot. A visible vessel or pigmented protuberance created from a vessel with a small attached clot has a rebleeding rate of 50% (Figs. 1–3 and 1–4). Active bleeding at endoscopy carries the highest rate of rebleeding at 70 to 80%. Mortality in patients with recurrent bleeding may be as high as 40%.[81]

Therapeutic Endoscopy: Injection Techniques

Variceal Injection Sclerosis Injection sclerosis for the treatment of esophageal varices, first reported in 1939,[82] was not popularized until the 1970s when fiberoptic flexible endoscopes became widely available. Sclerosing solutions are injected via a needle that is passed through the endoscope channel, allowing direct visualization of the index varix. It doesn't seem to matter whether the injections are made directly into or next to the varices, as long as hemostasis is achieved.[83,84] Commonly used sclerosants include the fatty acid derivatives morrhuate sodium and ethanolamine oleate, as well as synthetic oil compounds such as sodium tetradecyl sulfate and polydocanol, ethanol, and cyanoacrylate. These agents cause a necroinflammatory response resulting in thrombosis and fibrosis. Unwanted side effects include local ulcerations, fever, chest pain, bacteremia, pleural effusion, and, rarely, esophageal stricture.[85] The concentrations and amounts injected per site and per sclerotherapy session vary considerably, and there is no consensus as to the optimal technique.[86] Acute hemorrhage is controlled in 75 to 100% of patients with bleeding esophageal varices who receive sclerotherapy plus pharmacotherapy, in comparison with those who receive balloon tamponade with or without pharmacotherapy where control of hemorrhage is less successful (Fig. 1–5).[87–90] Repeat treatments are continued until varices are completely sclerosed. Intervals are usually set at 1–2 weeks to allow sclerosis site ulcerations to heal, while ensuring compliance and limiting the at-risk time for rebleeding. Bleeding risk correlates with variceal size and stage of cirrhosis, with larger varices and

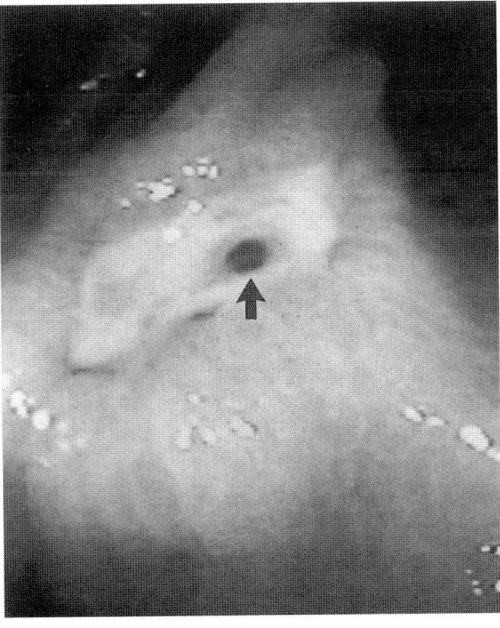

Figure 1–1 An atrophic vessel (*arrow*) in an ulcer crater appearing as a flat red spot. Therapy for *Helicobacter pylori* was prescribed. (See color plate 1–1.)

CHAPTER 1 · GASTROINTESTINAL BLEEDING

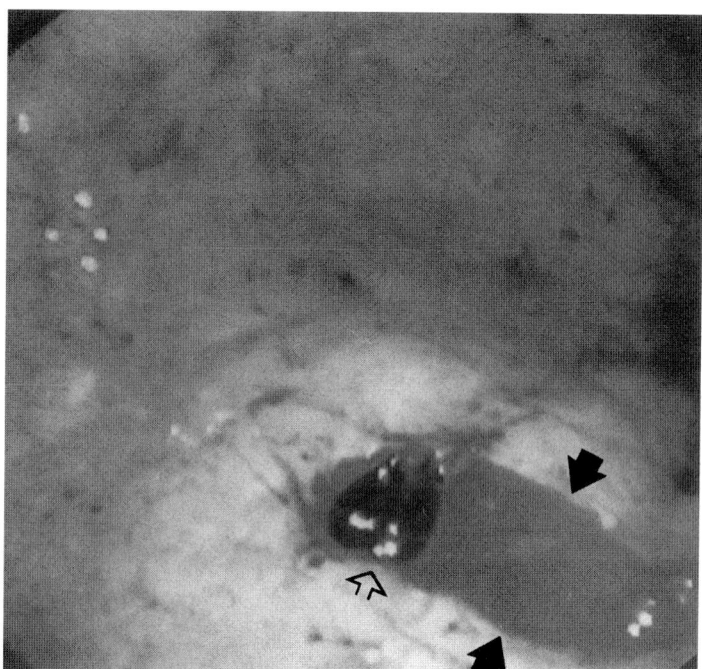

Figure 1–2 Active bleeding (*arrows*) from the base of a black clot (*open arrow*) obscuring an ulcer. Injection therapy was successful. (See color plate 1–2.)

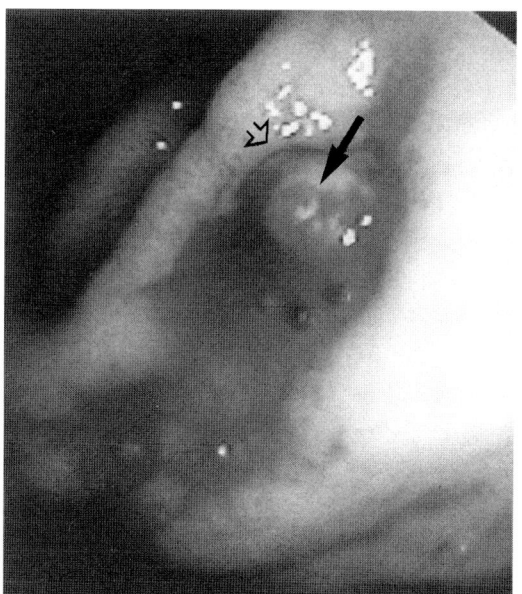

Figure 1–3 Visible vessel (*arrow*) with surrounding edematous folds (*open arrow*) from injection therapy. Rebleeding did not occur. (See color plate 1–3.)

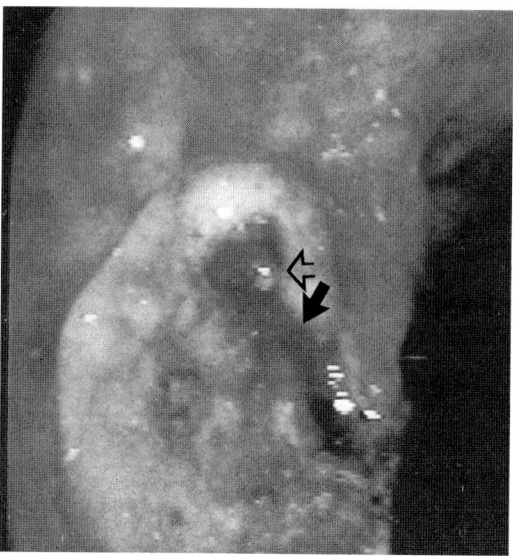

Figure 1–4 Minimal bleeding (*arrow*) from a pigmented protuberance (*open arrow*) in a large antral ulcer. Injection therapy halted further bleeding. (See color plate 1–4.)

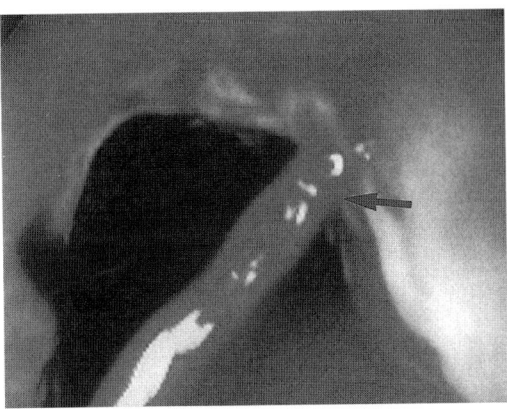

Figure 1–5 Active hemorrhage (*arrow*) from an esophageal varix seen only after rolling the patient to position the varix above the air-blood level. Sclerotherapy stopped the acute bleeding. (See color plate 1–5.)

Child C patients having predictably higher portal pressures, higher hepatic venous pressure gradients, and higher rates of variceal hemorrhage.[91] Sclerotherapy is clearly superior to no treatment for the prevention of rebleeding,[92–94] but it does not reduce portal pressure. The rebleeding risk between sclerotherapy sessions is 40 to 50%, compared with 70% or higher without any therapy. It is important to combine pharmacologic therapy with sclerotherapy to maximally reduce portal pressure medically while obliterating varices at risk for hemorrhage with sclerotherapy.[32,94] Even after varices are endoscopically ablated, surveillance endoscopies should be performed, as varices may recur unless definitive lowering of portal pressure has occurred. Injection therapy for bleeding gastric varices is performed less often for many reasons. Although proven to be present in 75% of patients studied by portal vein catheterization,[95] gastric varices are made visible by endoscopy in less than 10% of patients with portal hypertension (Fig. 1–6).[96] Their bleeding incidence is highly variable, and bleeding is more difficult to control with medical therapy, tamponade, or injection therapy. This is probably related to their larger size and higher intravariceal pressure. Injecting larger volumes of sclerosant per varix has increased the successful control of active bleeding.[97] Several recent trials using the tissue "superglue" isobutyl-2-cyanoacrylate have shown 93 to 100% control of acute gastric variceal bleeding;[98–100] isobutyl-2-cynnoacrylate immediately polymerizes upon contact with blood to form a tough adherent clot. Follow-up elective sclerotherapy for obliteration of gastric varices is unusual; transjugular intrahepatic portosystemic stent shunting (TIPSS), surgical shunting, or liver transplantation is most often recommended after gastric variceal hemorrhage, except in some cases of isolated gastric varices caused by splenic vein thrombosis wherein splenectomy is recommended.

Injection Therapy for Visible Vessels and Mucosal Tears Endoscopic injection therapy for bleeding peptic ulcers significantly reduces rebleeding, transfusion requirements, and need for urgent surgery compared with medical therapy alone.[101] Injection techniques have been used for all types of vessels (arteries and veins) seen or suspected at nearby areas of visible oozing blood. Medicinal agents used to treat bleeding sites include absolute or diluted ethanol, normal saline, hypertonic saline, dilute epinephrine at 1:10,000 or 1:20,000, concentrated dextrose solutions, sodium tetradecyl sulfate, polydocanol (or other typical sclerosants), and combinations of these. Trials comparing efficacy using different agents show overall little difference, suggesting that tamponade alone may be the mechanism responsible for cessation of bleeding. Collectively, these agents are about 80% effective at initially controlling bleeding, with 20 to 30% recurrent bleeding usually occurring within 48 hours.[81] When bleeding is massive or the patient presents with shock, a large bleeding artery is likely responsible.[102] Several studies suggest that using a sclerosing agent for definitive obliteration of the artery is effective for the prevention of rebleeding.[103–105] In dogs with experimentally induced ulcers, ethanol and polydocanol, but not epinephrine, caused definite arteriolar thrombosis.[106] Ethanol and tetradecyl together resulted in the most effective mesenteric artery sclerosis but also

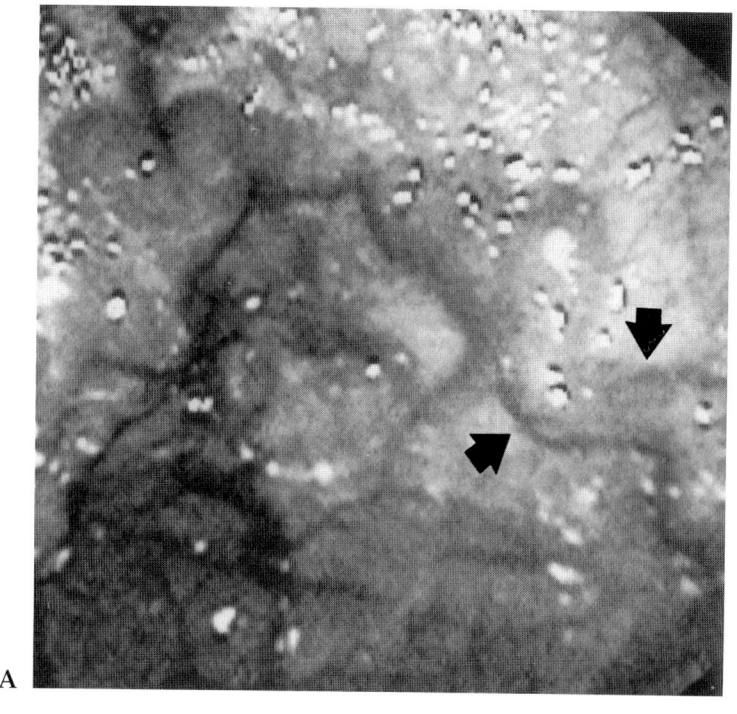

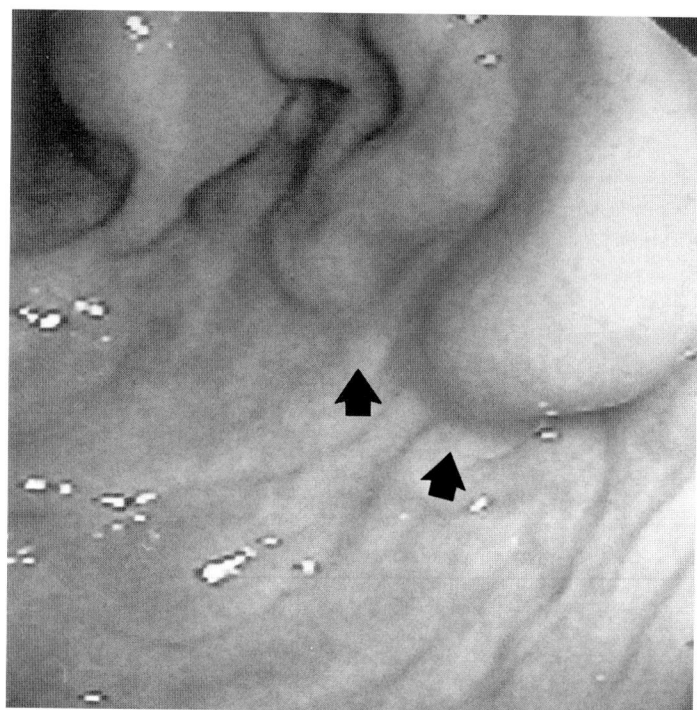

Figure 1–6 (A) Dark gastric varices (*arrows*) are easily recognized as veins compared with (B). (B) Light-colored gastric varices (*arrows*) may be overlooked as prominent rugae. (See color plate 1–6.)

caused significant transmural damage.[107] Most endoscopists will safely inject 20 to 30 mL of dilute epinephrine circumferentially around vessels and then inject small amounts of a sclerosant directly into the vessel. Absolute ethanol should be used in 0.1- to 0.2-mL increments per injection site, not exceeding 1 to 2 mL total, to reduce the risk of transmural injury and the potential for perforation. Sclerosing agents may not be advisable for use in thin-walled areas, such as the duodenum or right colon. Advantages of injection therapy include low cost, relatively easy mastery of the technique, and low complication rates. Many endoscopists are combining injection therapy with hemostatic therapies, such as thermal coagulation. In a controlled trial, this combination was proven safe and effective,[108] but its superiority over injection therapy or thermal coagulation alone has not been established. Randomized studies are needed to determine the optimal combinations associated with minimal risk and cost.

Thermal Coagulation Techniques

Monopolar, Bipolar, and Heater Probe Devices Tissue cutting or coagulation results from heat generated when high-frequency current is passed through tissues that resist its flow. Monopolar circuits consist of current produced by a generator and flowing to an active electrode, through the patient, to a distant return electrode (grounding pad), and then back to the generator. In bipolar or multipolar circuits, the distance between the electrodes is minute, with current flowing through a very small amount of tissue. This allows for the use of lower pressure settings with less potential for complications. Therefore, most thermal coagulation probes in use today for endoscopic hemostasis are multipolar.[109] Heater probes are computer-controlled thermal cautery devices set to deliver the desired amount of energy to a tip coated with a non-stick surface.[110] The resulting tissue effect is essentially the same as with multipolar probes. Several randomized controlled trials have shown that thermal coagulation of bleeding or visible vessels is efficacious at controlling hemorrhage and decreasing rebleeding.[111–113] Depth of coagulation with the larger 3.2-mm probes varies with watt setting, tissue contact time, and applied pressure.[114] High-power settings theoretically cut off the current when the tissue temperature reaches 100° C, as water vaporizes and dehydrated tissue conducts heat poorly.[115] Presence of desiccating tissue may also result in a larger hole in the vessel wall and exacerbation of bleeding. The optimal technique is to coapt opposing sides of the vessel wall by pushing firmly with the larger 3.2-mm probes and then slowly heat using low-power settings (15 to 25 W) with longer (10 seconds) contact times.[114] Randomized trials comparing multipolar coagulation to laser, injection therapy, and heater probe have shown equivalent efficacy for hemostasis of bleeding peptic ulcers.[116–119] Heater probes and multipolar thermal coagulation techniques have also been used for treatment of bleeding due to Mallory-Weiss tears, Dieulafoy's lesion (Fig. 1–7), vascular angiomata, postsphincterotomy and postpolypectomy hemorrhage, watermelon stomach, and postirradiation-induced mucosal hemorrhage.[112,120–125] Although low-power settings are optimal for these applications as well, care must be taken in

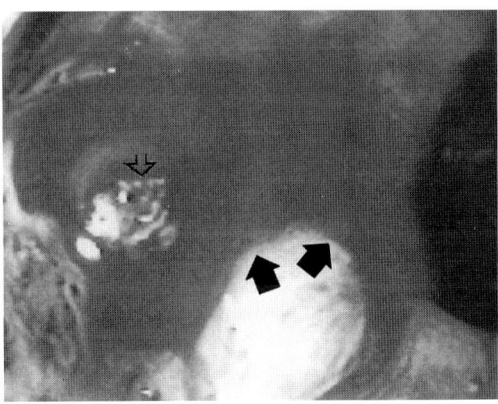

Figure 1–7 Blood (*arrows*) oozing from a Dieulafoy's lesion (*open arrow*). Thermal coagulation was successful. (See color plate 1–7.)

thin-walled areas to tailor the pressure and tissue contact time to minimize the potential for perforation. A meta-analysis of 25 randomized controlled trials comparing the efficacy of thermocoagulation or injection therapy with that of nonendoscopic management for bleeding peptic ulcers revealed significantly reduced rebleeding, decreased need for surgery, and 30% reduction in mortality in patients treated with endoscopic therapy.[126]

Laser Endoscopic injection therapy and heater probe or multipolar thermal coagulation techniques are used most often for the management of acute upper GI bleeding because they are relatively inexpensive, effective, and portable. Laser therapy is more expensive and more difficult to master but very effective for all types of bleeding lesions. By 1973, it became feasible to pass both argon and neodymium:yttrium-aluminum-garnet (Nd:-YAG) laser energy through fiberoptic gastroscopes.[127,128] Laser light is aimed at bleeding sites, with a plastic catheter waveguide placed through the endoscope channel. Laser energy is selectively absorbed by the red color of hemoglobin, giving this method a theoretical advantage in controlling hemorrhage. Photons of light that are absorbed or scattered at the tissue surface produce heat. The amount of heat produced depends on the laser type and tissue exposure time. Tissue absorbs light of different wavelengths at various degrees; therefore, the argon, Nd:YAG, and CO_2 lasers produce tissue coagulation to different depths. Because of its capacity to coagulate to a depth of 5 mm as well as produce a wider (circumferential) tissue effect from immediate scatter, the Nd:YAG laser is employed most often for gastrointestinal hemostasis. For optimal use, the recommendation is to use short pulses (0.5 to 1 second) of relatively high energy (60 to 90 J) in a tight circle immediately surrounding the bleeding site and aimed directly at the point of last bleeding.[129] By 1990, the largest uncontrolled study of the use of Nd:YAG laser in 1058 patients with bleeding peptic ulcers showed that hemostasis was achieved in 94%, with a complication rate from perforation of less than 2%.[130] Multiple randomized controlled trials comparing Nd:YAG laser with other forms of endoscopic hemostasis for peptic ulcer reveal a slight benefit of laser to other methods.[131–133] Meta-analysis of trials of laser photocoagulation versus control for bleeding ulcers favored laser for significantly reducing rebleeding, controlling acute bleeding, reducing the need for surgery, and reducing mortality.[134] Laser therapy has also been used in many patients to control acute and chronic bleeding from angiomata, telangiectasis in Osler-Weber-Rendu disease, and watermelon stomach.[135–138]

Argon Plasma Coagulation Argon plasma coagulation is a noncontact thermal technique that combines the technologies of monopolar electrocoagulation and laser photocoagulation. It is portable, easy to use, and less expensive than the Nd:YAG laser. Argon gas flows through a catheter as a spray on the target tissue surface, with transmission of the high-frequency electrical current to the gas by a thin electric wire at the tip of the catheter. This allows for rapid thermal treatment of a large surface area, with a maximum depth of coagulation at 3 to 4 mm.[139] Trials with this therapy in patients with a variety of GI bleeding lesions revealed excellent hemostasis and safety.[140,141]

Mechanical Techniques
Endoscopic Clips Metallic clips for endoscopic hemostasis were first introduced in Japan in 1975.[142] These devices are most useful when the exact site of bleeding is visible. As there is essentially no damage to surrounding tissues, endoclip devices are ideal for thin-walled segments of the GI tract, such as a protruding artery in the base of a deep duodenal ulcer or bleeding from postpolypectomy sites. Studies comparing the use of hemoclips with other hemostatic therapies showed no significant difference in efficacy.[143,144]

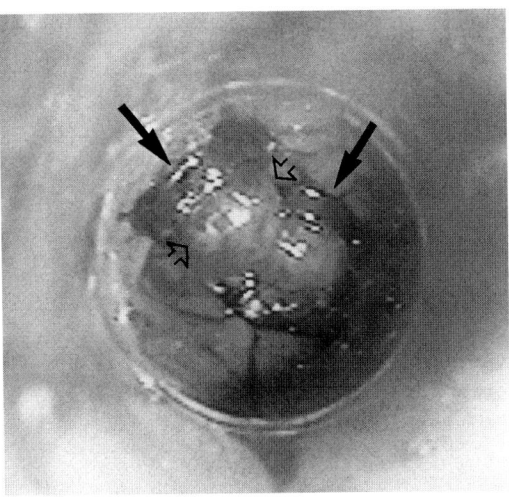

Figure 1–8 Endoscopic view after deploying multiple rubber bands (*arrows*) on esophageal varices (*open arrows*). (See color plate 1–8.)

Band Ligation Band ligation for the treatment of esophageal varices was first introduced in 1988.[145] Today band ligation has exceeded injection sclerosis as the primary method of elective endoscopic treatment for esophageal varices (Fig. 1–8). Compared with injection sclerosis, band ligation is as effective but associated with fewer complications of infection, esophageal stricture, and site ulceration.[146,119] Band ligation has also been used to control bleeding attributed to vascular angiomata, Dieulafoy's lesion, Mallory-Weiss tears, and peptic ulcers.[150–152]

Endoscopic Tattooing Unusual lesions, such as Dieulafoy's lesion or other lesions that are difficult to access and require subsequent endoscopic or surgical therapy, can be tattooed at the initial endoscopy to aid in their relocation. India ink diluted with 1:10 or 1:100 saline can be autoclaved or passed through a microfilter[153] prior to use. It is injected in increments of 0.1 to 0.5 mL at or circumferentially around lesions and later can be seen on either the gut mucosal or the serosal surface.[154–155] Ink tattoos remain in the tissues for years and are considered permanent.[156]

Radiologic Diagnosis and Management

Nuclear Scintigraphy

Nuclear GI scintigraphy may be helpful in patients with obscure GI bleeding. Most often, patients have already had one or more endoscopic evaluations with negative findings. A typical scenario is an elderly person without abdominal pain who intermittently experiences melena or passage of maroon-colored stools. Lesions may be anywhere from the nasal mucosa to the right colon. Vascular angiomata are a common source of bleeding in this setting,[10,157,158] whereas duodenal or jejunal diverticuli, neoplasias, hemobilia, or other lesions are less likely. A small bowel enteroscopic examination would ideally be used for diagnosis and coagulation therapy. However, if such an examination is unavailable or nondiagnostic, nuclear scintigraphy may be beneficial (Fig. 1–9A, 9B).

Labeling a patient's red blood cells with technetium pertechnetate allows for immediate and delayed scanning; the tracer remains sufficiently detectable for about 24 hours. Bleeding rates as low as 0.1 to 0.5 mL/min (one half to two units packed red blood cells/24 h) can be detected.[159] Technetium 99–labeled sulfur colloid injected intravenously is followed by immediate scanning and hence is limited to patients with active bleeding. In the clinical setting, nuclear scintigraphy can identify bleeding with 40 to 65% sensitivity and 25% specificity. Low specificity is explained by dispersion of the tracer once it has extravasated into the gut lumen.

Angiography

Angiography is an excellent adjunct to both diagnosis and treatment of brisk GI bleeding. It is usually employed when standard diagnostic endoscopies are nondiagnostic or therapeutically unsuccessful

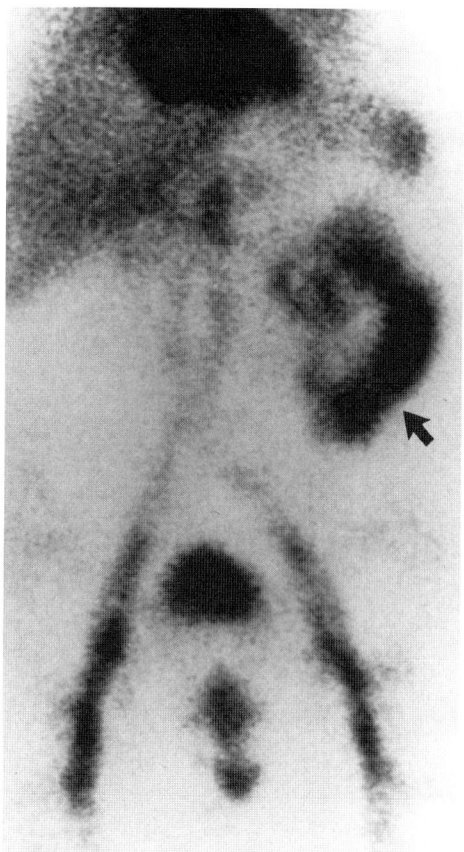
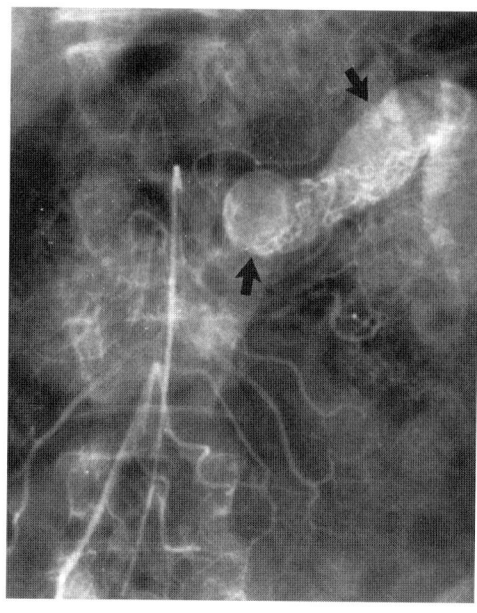

Figure 1–9 This patient had recurrent GI hemorrhage with a nondiagnostic endoscopic exam. **(A)** A tagged red cell study revealed extravasation of radiotracer into the proximal jejunum (*arrow*). **(B)** Angiogram of the superior mesenteric artery demonstrates pooling of contrast in a long segment of jejunal wall (*arrows*). At laparotomy, a large diffuse cavernous hemangioma was resected.

(Fig. 1–10). Although most helpful in cases of voluminous lower GI bleeding, where colonoscopic visualization of the mucosa is markedly impaired, many rapidly bleeding upper GI lesions escaping endoscopic control can be managed with angiography. Selective celiac and superior mesenteric artery catheterization outlines the arterial supply of the distal duodenum and proximal jejunum. Superselection of smaller arteries with microcatheters and steerable wires allows for localization of very distal bleeding arterial branches. The formerly popular agent vasopressin with its potent arteriolar smooth-muscle constricting effect is used less frequently now due to the unwanted systemic side effects, which include reduced renal and mesenteric blood flow, coronary ischemia, myocardial infarction, and arrhythmias.[160]

Angiographic evaluation can be tailored for a specific site if a nuclear medicine study indicates a distinct focus of bleeding. This, however, does not exclude the possibility of a second GI bleed, although that is statistically less likely. If no distinct focus of bleeding is predetermined from either nuclear medicine or endoscopic studies, then a full mesenteric evaluation is necessary.

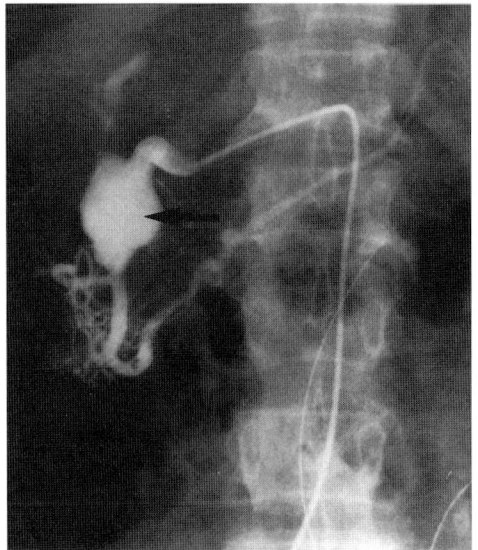

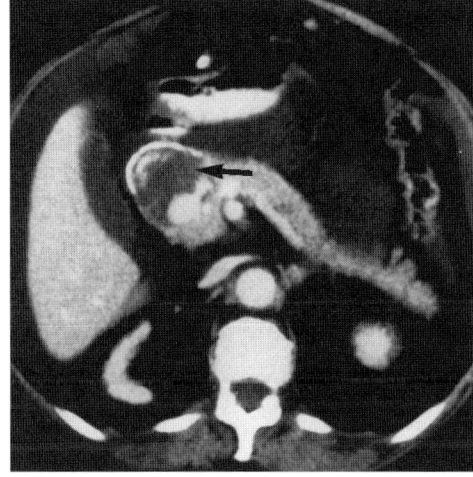

Figure 1–10 This patient had recurrent upper GI bleeding without visible lesions on endoscopy. **(A)** Celiac axis injection demonstrated a pseudoaneurysm (*arrow*) of the gastroduodenal artery. **(B)** CT image of the pseudoaneurysm revealed partial thrombosis (*arrow*). The pseudoaneurysm was successfully resected without complication.

Bleeding is classified as being either upper or lower GI in origin. Upper GI bleeding evaluation begins with a celiac arteriogram. The left gastric branch of the celiac artery should be of particular interest given its supply to the stomach, as should be the gastric duodenal artery, which is commonly involved in duodenal ulcerations. If no source of bleeding is identified, then the next vessel for study should be the superior mesenteric artery (SMA), followed by the inferior mesenteric artery (IMA); these are the primary vessels involved in lower GI bleeding. It has been recommended that, prior to IMA angiography, limited aortography be performed because atherosclerotic disease at this level may make catheterization of this vessel risky.

When evaluating the mesenteric vessels, prolonged imaging is of paramount importance for detecting any staining or blush, which may represent a hemorrhage. Recognizing a bleed can be difficult with subtraction images, secondary to bowel motion. Glucagon can be used to help decrease peristalsis prior to filming. Also, the images can be viewed in the nonsubtracted mode. An alternative to conventional contrast, CO_2 angiography is being discussed as an approach to GI bleeding. Being less viscous then iodinated contrast, CO_2 easily traverses hemorrhagic vessels and expands as it becomes extravascular, allowing easier visualization.

Most physicians familiar with mesenteric examinations understand that these are often low-yield studies because the patient is not actively bleeding during the study. The bleeding rates required for visibility on corrective arteriograms have often been quoted as about 0.5 mL/min for an upper GI bleed and 1 mL/min for a lower GI bleed.[161] Recent studies have used provocative testing in the form of urokinase and heparin to help initiate active bleeding at the time of the angiogram. This has been done with both direct and systemic infusion of urokinase and heparin followed by contrast evaluation.[162,163] Although it may seem unusual to deliberately incite an active bleed, an argument can be made that it is even more risky to have a patient with a massive GI bleed in an outpatient setting rather than in a controlled hospital situation.

Upper GI bleeding secondary to varices and portal hypertension are evaluated and managed differently. Treatment often involves TIPSS or surgical decompression, as will be discussed later.

Interventional Therapy for GI Bleed
Classically, transcatheter control of upper GI bleeding has been obtained with the use of vasopressin, with an initial dose of 0.2 U/min regardless of which vessel was being treated (Fig. 1–11). After 20 minutes, arteriography is repeated, and if there is no further bleeding the catheter is left in place and the patient placed on a continuous infusion of 0.2 U/min for 24 hours. The patient is reevaluated after 24 hours and the dose of vasopressin is reduced to 0.1 U/min. This is continued for 24 hours and again the patient is reevaluated. If no further bleeding is noted, then normal saline is infused for an additional 12 hours, at which time the patient is reevaluated and the catheter removed if all has normalized.

If the initial 0.2 U/min vasopressin dose does not control the bleeding, the dose is increased to 0.4 U/min, with an angiogram obtained 20 minutes after initiation of this dose. If there is no further hemorrhage, then the catheter is left in place and the dose tapered over 48 to 72 hours. If the 0.4-U, dose is not sufficient, then embolization therapy ("embotherapy") is performed at this point or the patient is taken to surgery.

Embolization Therapy
Embolotherapy has emerged as the preferred arteriographic method to control bleeding GI lesions (Fig. 1–12). Advantages over vasoconstrictors include more definitive control of bleeding and fewer potential complications. Gelfoam is the most widely

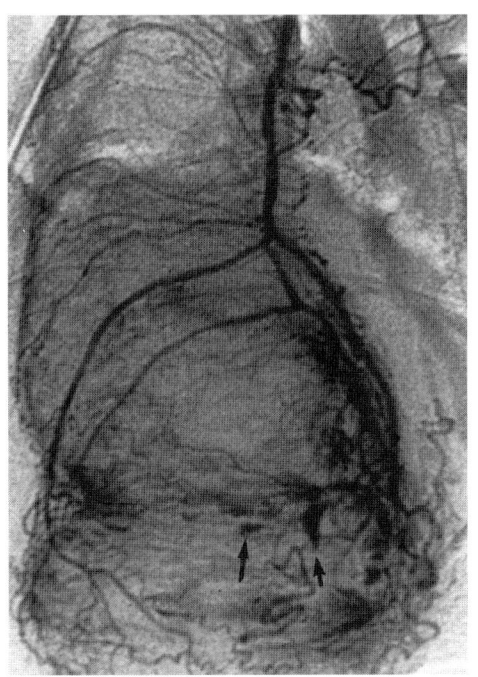
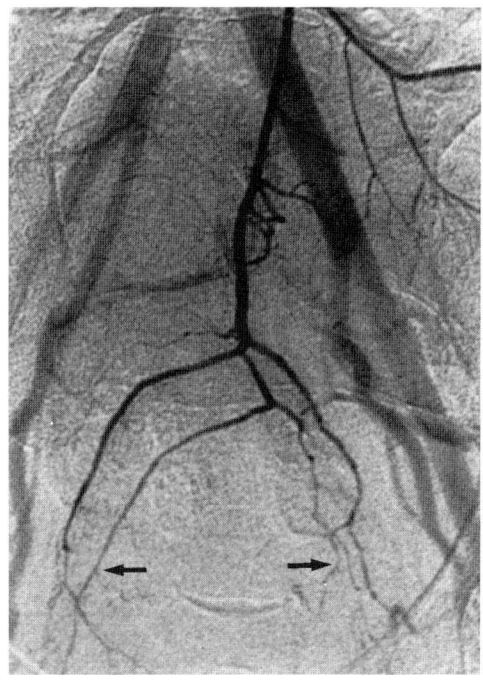

Figure 1–11 Despite endoscopic therapy, this HIV-positive patient had continued bleeding from multiple rectal ulcers. **(A)** An inferior mesenteric artery angiogram demonstrates several discrete areas of contrast pooling in the rectal vault (*arrows*). Vasopressin was infused at 0.2 U/min for 20 minutes, then stopped. **(B)** No further extravasation of contrast was seen; vasoconstriction of end arterioles was evident (*arrows*).

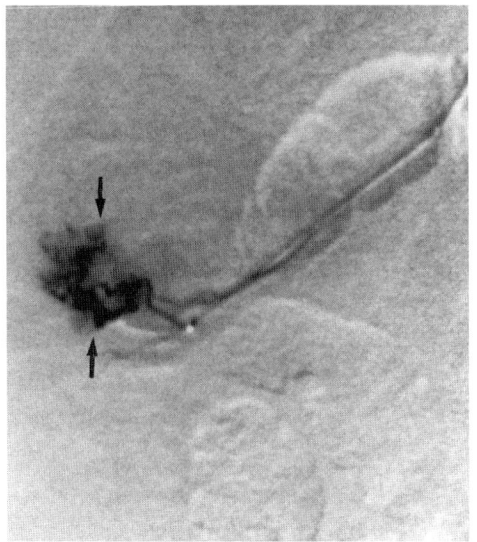 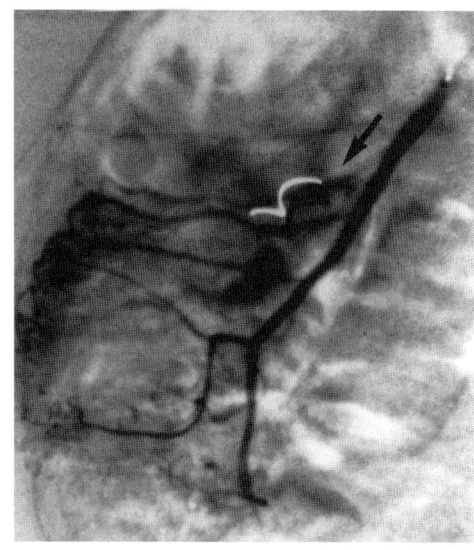

Figure 1–12 **(A)** A patient with lower GI bleeding and high surgical risk underwent angiography with superselection of a right colonic branch demonstrating a bleeding angiodysplasia (*arrows*). **(B)** Angiogram following coil embolization (*arrow*) showed no further contrast extravasation.

used resorbable agent; it is recommended that large particles be used to avoid occlusion of the smaller mucosal arteries, which can result in tissue ischemia, necrosis, and infraction.[164] Resorbable materials are usually chosen when the cause of bleeding is benign; recanalization of the vessel occurs after several weeks, with the potential for rebleeding. Bleeding from malignant causes or from larger arteries requires permanent embolization. Materials used include polyvinyl alcohol (PVA), absolute ethanol, cyanoacrylic glues, and platinum coils.

If bleeding is emanating from a gastric source, the bleeding site will be supplied by the left gastric artery in 85% of cases.[165] Mucosal oozing lesions, such as from Mallory-Weiss tears or diffuse gastritis, can be effectively controlled with infusion of vasopressin into the left gastric artery.[166] Rebleeding occurs in up to 25% of patients.[167,168] Due to the rich anastomotic supply to the stomach, sacrifice of this vessel can usually be done without adverse outcome. Even when a source of bleeding is not seen in an upper GI lesion, certain authors have advocated prophylactic embolization of the vessel.[163] The embolic agent of choice in the left gastric artery is Gelfoam pledgets, although stainless steel coils are often placed in conjunction with Gelfoam and/or as standalone embolic agents.

The duodenum is supplied by branches of the pancreaticoduodenal arcade and the gastroduodenal artery. Bleeding lesions usually result from ulcer penetration into one of the smaller branches of the gastroduodenal artery, and embolization of this artery usually stops acute bleeding. Proximal and distal control of the bleed is required, possibly necessitating embolization of the inferior pancreaticoduodenal arcade.[169] Hemobilia may occur posttrauma, postcholecystectomy, postpercutaneous transhepatic drainage, or in association with hepatobiliary malignancy.[170] Although tagged red cell scanning, computed tomography (CT), and endoscopic retrograde cholangiography may point to potential bleeding sources, hepatic arteriography has the advantage of definitively localizing the bleeding.[171]

Superselective hepatic artery occlusion for control of bleeding can usually be performed without causing significant liver ischemia owing to the rich supply of portal blood to the liver. Portal patency can be established by delayed SMA angiography, ultrasonography, or CT, and is critical information prior to hepatic artery embolization. Administration of prophylactic broad-spectrum antibiotics has been recommended to prevent sepsis or hepatic abscess.[171]

Regardless of the embolic agent, two issues are critical to bowel embolization: (1) gaining proximal and distal control of the bleeding vessel and (2) avoiding reflux. The importance of both proximal and distal control of a bleeding vessel is obvious. This is particularly important when considering a duodenal ulcer that is supplied by the gastric duodenal artery. Occluding only the proximal source simply causes blood to reflux through the arcuate vessels from the SMA. Separately, the issue of reflux is generally less of a problem with coils than with Gelfoam, PVA, or sclerosing agents such as ethanol. Constant fluoroscopic monitoring and a nonrushed approach will help prevent this potential complication.

TIPSS for Portal Hypertensive Bleeding

TIPSS has become a popular method for salvaging patients with portal hypertensive bleeding not controlled by endoscopic therapy.[172–174] The mortality for any Childs class is lower for TIPSS than for urgent surgery in this setting. As a successfully placed TIPSS definitively lowers portal pressure,[175] rebleeding post TIPSS is significantly lower than in patients treated with endoscopic sclerotherapy or band ligation. The incidence of rebleeding between endoscopic sessions is about 50%. Three of four prospective randomized studies revealed a reduced incidence of rebleeding with TIPSS compared to sclerotherapy, suggesting that TIPSS be considered as primary therapy for the prevention of rebleeding in patients with portal hypertension.[176–179] A concern about TIPSS, however, is for the promotion or worsening of hepatic encephalopathy due to the shunting of blood flow from an already impaired liver. Hepatic encephalopathy occurs in about 5% of Childs A patients, 10 to 15% of Childs B patients, and about 25% of Childs C patients who undergo TIPSS. If the encephalopathy is debilitating or uncontrollable with medical therapy, the TIPSS can be occluded, reversing the encephalopathy. Chronic hemolysis may occur in up to 10% of patients, presumably from fragmentation of erythrocytes flowing against and through the mesh stent.[180–181] After endothelialization occurs, hemolysis should abate. Like endoscopic variceal ablation, patients who have undergone TIPSS require close follow-up and maintenance to ensure that their shunt remains functional.[182] Most occluded stents can be successfully revised. Early stent occlusion is usually due to thrombosis, and phenprocoumon[183] or another anticoagulant may decrease the incidence of this complication. Chronic or late shunt stenosis due to pseudointimal hyperplasia occurs in 50% of patients by 1 year. During TIPSS, transient biliary venous fistulae may be responsible for promoting this obliterative process.[184]

TIPSS-Induced Renal, Humoral, and Cardiovascular Changes

Although the hemodynamic effects of TIPSS are not completely understood, shunting an estimated 20% of systemic blood flow directly into the right heart in patients who already have a hyperdynamic circulation may ultimately prove damaging to the heart and lungs.[185–186] Therefore, patients with known significant right heart failure or pulmonary hypertension should not undergo TIPSS, although the degree of heart or lung dysfunction precluding TIPSS is unknown. The augmented preload with TIPSS results in increased atrionatriuretic peptide release, increased renal blood flow, and decreased renin and angiotensin levels. Also, as blood is shunted away from the liver, hepatic sinusoidal pressure falls, resulting in decreased serum norepinephrine.

Although not completely understood, portal hypertension–induced impairment of renal proximal tubular sodium excretion may be related to selective vasoconstriction of renal arterioles via norepinephrine-stimulated endothelin effects. Post-TIPSS, as blood is shunted away from the liver, sinusoidal pressure is reduced, serum epinephrine levels fall, and, concomitantly, renal sodium excretion improves.[187–189] These physiologic alterations post-TIPSS may underlie the improved mortality in patients with hepatorenal syndrome who undergo TIPSS.[190] Transjugular intrahepatic portosytemic shunting has also been lifesaving in patients with symptomatic hepatic hydrothorax.[191,192] This complication occurs in less than 5% of patients with ascites; however, due to the negative intrathoracic pressure relative to intra-abdominal pressure, ascites is pulled into the chest through diaphragmatic defects and can result in tension hydrothorax or significantly impaired respiration.

To TIPSS or Not To TIPSS

Deciding who should receive an elective TIPSS as opposed to other therapy is difficult, requiring that careful attention be paid to the individual's hepatic function, cardiorespiratory status, as well as lifestyle, functional status, desired therapeutic goals, and eligibility for liver transplantation. Elective TIPSS appears most suitable for patients with recurrently bleeding esophageal or gastric varices and in whom liver transplantation may or may not be an option for the near future. The decision to perform a TIPSS in patients with medically refractory ascites for improvement of lifestyle must be weighed against the risk of causing further deterioration in liver function and increasing mortality.[193–195] Future development of covered stents or alternative materials to prolong shunt patency may also influence clinical use.

TIPSS: The Procedure in a Nutshell

Prior to the procedure, it is important to verify portal vein patency. This can be performed using ultrasonography, which will also tell whether or not ascites is present. Certain operators prefer to drain the ascites prior to the procedure as this makes the liver less mobile and makes it easier to pass a needle from the hepatic to the portal vein.

We have generally been able to perform TIPSS using conscious sedation rather than general anesthesia. The procedure begins with cannulation of the right internal jugular vein (although the left internal jugular vein can also be cannulated, should the right be occluded). We perform this under direct ultrasonographic guidance. Next, a long sheath is placed. These sheaths are included in any of the several prepackaged TIPSS kits. Next, we catheterize the right hepatic vein. It is important to take a few extra moments and verify that you are indeed within the right hepatic vein (Fig. 1–13A). This can be performed by angling the image intensifier laterally and verifying that the hepatic vein courses posteriorly. If you are within the middle hepatic vein by mistake, you will see your catheter, wire, or contrast course anteriorly. Once you have verified that you are within the right hepatic vein, intravascular pressures are stabilized. Some operators then perform a wedged hepatic angiogram using either a contrast or CO_2 to help delineate the portal vein via reflux through the hepatic sinusoids. There are others, however, who rely on landmarks only and use a blind puncture. There have been numerous methods described for detecting the portal vein from ultrasonography to direct percutaneous puncture prior to the actual TIPSS procedure. Regardless of how the portal vein is located, the theory is to place a Calopinto needle into the right hepatic vein approximately 2 cm proximal to the right hepatic vein/IVC origin and to direct the needle anteriorly and laterally, approximately 45 degrees to the patient, and to advance the needle approximately 1.5 to 2 cm per throw. A syringe is then connected to the Calopinto needle and blood is aspirated while the needle is brought back slowly. When blood is seen, contrast is

CHAPTER 1 · GASTROINTESTINAL BLEEDING

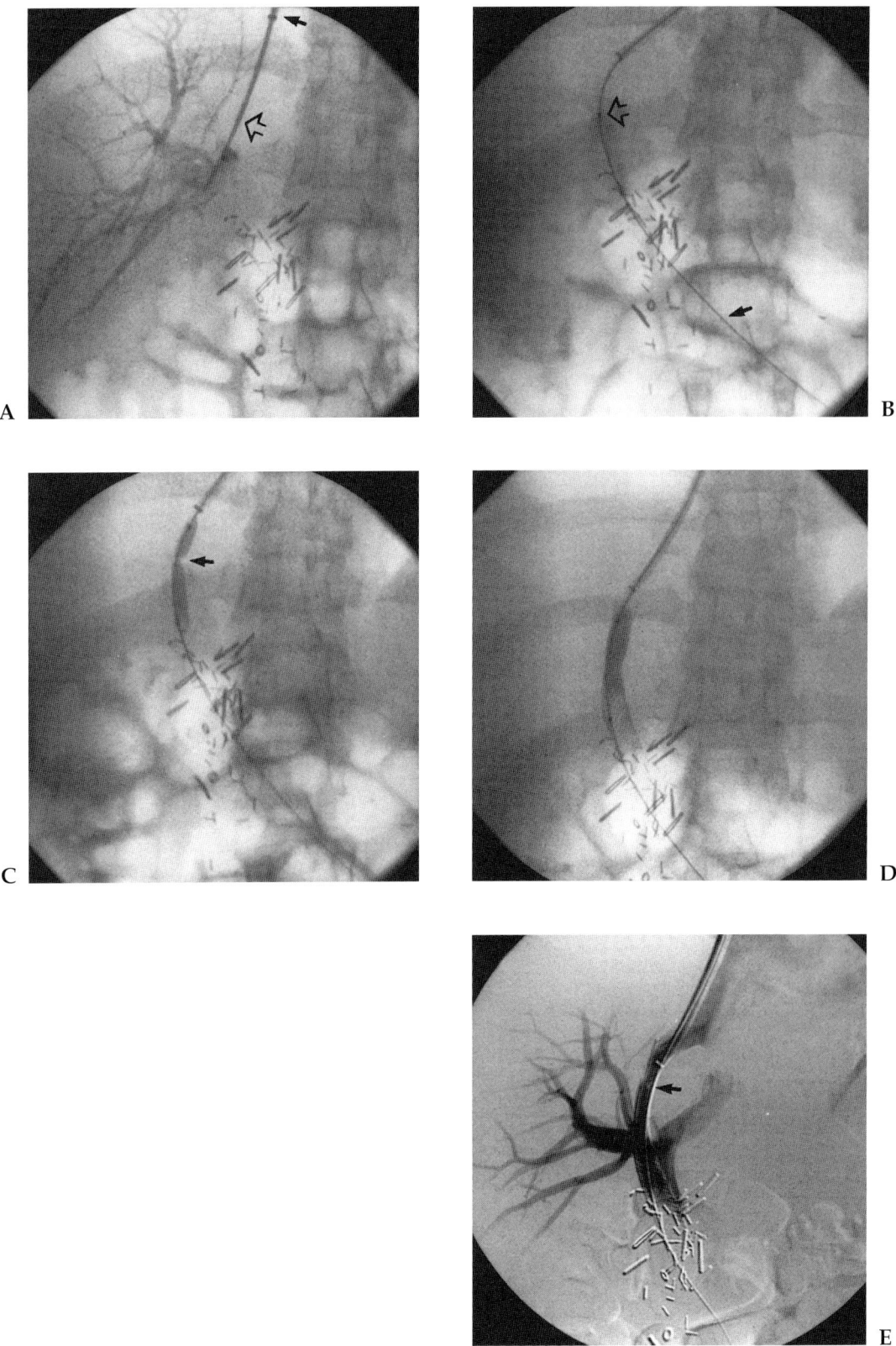

injected to verify its placement in the portal vein. Once the portal vein has been cannulated, a glide wire is placed, followed by a hockey-stick type of catheter. The Calopinto needle is removed during the course of this exchange and a stiffer wire replaces the glide wire (Fig. 1–13B). Pressures are obtained within the portal venous system at this time, although there usually is little doubt as to the presence of portal hypertension because these patients have often received various endoscopic and other procedures verifying the presence of varices. Contrast evaluation of the portal vein is then performed, with specific attention to the puncture site.

If the puncture site is adequate, the tract is balloon-dilated (Fig. 1–13C) and a 10- to 12-mm Wall stent placed in the tract (Fig. 1–13D). The stent should not be placed too deeply in the portal vein so as not to cause any difficulty for the surgeons when cross-clamping, should the patient be eligible for liver transplantation. Stents are placed to cover the full tract, including the area adjacent to the hepatic vein, which is often the area most difficult to keep patent (Fig. 1–13E). After these have been placed, initial dilatation of the stents to 8 mm is performed, with pressures reevaluated in both the portal and hepatic circulations. It desirable to leave a pressure gradient less than 12 mm Hg. Subsequent dilatations can be performed to obtain the proper gradient, keeping in mind that there is always a trade-off between bleeding and encephalopathy with these patients. After the tract has been adequately dilated, we remove all lines and sheaths and keep the patient's head off the bed and elevated 30 degrees for a few hours post procedure. The following morning the patient undergoes baseline hepatic ultrasonography with flow evaluation through the shunt, with routine (every 3 months) ultrasonographic follow-up to preempt any stent occlusion or significant stenosis.

Surgical Management

Historical and Epidemiologic Considerations

The availability of therapeutic endoscopy, understanding of the importance of *H. pylori* eradication for peptic ulcer disease, and improvements in acid-suppressive therapy have collectively resulted in a marked reduction in the use of surgery for bleeding peptic ulcer. Formerly, ulcers recurred after initial healing in 70% of patients, and those who rebled predictably did so within 3 years.[196] Surgery was classically recommended for patients with recurrent bleeding ulcers. Today, with antibiotic eradication of *H. pylori* infection, ulcers recur in only a minority of cases (4%). Ulcer rebleeding rates also declined.[56,57] Because many combinations of 1- to 2-week antibiotic regimens for *H. pylori* eradication are effective, surgery for *H. pylori*-associated ulceration will predictably become rare. Chronic use of H_2- receptor antagonists or

Figure 1–13 (A) Calopinto needle is shown entering the portal venous system (*open arrow*). The vascular sheath is seen in the region of the hepatic vein–inferior vena cava junction (*arrow*). (B) A wire has been placed into the portal venous system (*arrow*) followed by placement of an angioplasty balloon for hepatic parenchymal dilatation (*open arrow*). (C) Balloon dilatation between the hepatic vein and the portal vein is performed. The area of highest stenosis is at the area just distal to the hepatic vein puncture site (*arrow*). (D) A Wall stent has been placed across the newly formed tract and is being subsequently dilated with an angioplasty balloon. (E) A second stent has been added to further bridge the stenotic regions seen on angioplasty (*arrow*). Contrast injection now shows a patent tract between the portal vein and the inferior vena cava.

proton pump inhibitors also reduces recurrent ulcer bleeding,[197] but their cost and poor patient compliance with chronic prophylactic medical therapy renders surgery a valuable alternative approach to non–H. pylori-associated bleeding peptic ulcers.

Who Should Receive an Operation, and When?

Studies of the anatomy of bleeding ulcers reveal that the majority occur as a result of erosion of an ulcer into medium-sized arteries in the submucosa[102] and therefore should be amenable to control with endoscopic techniques. Lesser curvature ulcers eroding into the left gastric artery, or posteroduodenal ulcers eroding into the gastroduodenal artery represent a minority of cases that most often require surgery for definitive therapy.[198] In other cases, failure to initially obtain hemostasis endoscopically occurs secondary to inaccessibility of the bleeding vessel or torrential hemorrhage. These patients are generally referred for emergency operative management, with attendant mortality rates of 7 to 15%.[199,200,202] The risk for and management of recurrent bleeding after initial endoscopic hemostasis of gastric and duodenal ulcers are less well defined. A number of factors have been identified as placing the patient at high risk for recurrent bleeding, including shock, ulcer larger than 2 cm, hemoglobin level less than 7.9, endoscopic stigmata of recent bleed (nonbleeding visible vessel, adherent clot on the ulcer base), and obesity.[198–201] Shock is the best predictor for recurrent bleeding,[30–203] and rebleeding in the hospital carries a 6- to 12-fold increase in mortality.[204] Patients with shock are best candidates for early (urgent) operative intervention to prevent their highly predictable rebleeding and morbid or mortal outcome. Prospective studies comparing early surgery to conservative therapy and defining the specific criteria for early surgery have yielded impressively low mortality rates of 0 to 7%.[205–207] Although the specific criteria varied among these studies, they commonly included early surgery for patient age greater than 60, shock at presentation, initial transfusion requirements in excess of 6 U of blood, or total blood and colloid requirements within 48 hours in excess of 12 U. The only prospective randomized trial looking specifically at timing of surgery in acute bleeding ulcers has been criticized for its small patient sample, for encompassing several types of operations, and for inequalities in patient characteristics (ages, degrees of underlying diseases).[208] However, it revealed a low (7%) mortality in elderly (older than 60) patients who underwent early surgery, as opposed to a 43% operative mortality for those undergoing delayed surgical management. In a separate study of 5112 patients with bleeding ulcers, 3.5% underwent emergency surgery, with a surgical mortality rate of 12% and an overall mortality of 4.5%.[209] Surgery was performed for active bleeding from an unidentified upper GI site, bleeding uncontrolled by endoscopic methods, total transfusion requirements in excess of 8 U of blood, or rebleeding with hypotension, tachycardia, hematemesis, or melena. Although not a randomized study, the overall low mortality in this large group of bleeding patients points out the logic in identifying and implementing selection criteria for surgical intervention. A large prospective randomized trial has been conducted comparing the repeat endoscopic treatment to surgery for patients with peptic ulcer bleeding. This study did not show an increase in mortality rate for repeat endoscopic hemostasis, even if the second attempt failed and the patient underwent salvage surgery. It did identify hypotension at randomization and ulcer size at least 2 cm as independent factors likely to result in endoscopic failure.[210] A retrospective analysis of a larger patient cohort revealed a higher mortality rate among those patients undergoing surgery as opposed to repeat endoscopic management; however, risk factors for mortality included age and number of concomitant diseases, malignant disease, rebleeding episodes, and surgical complications.[211]

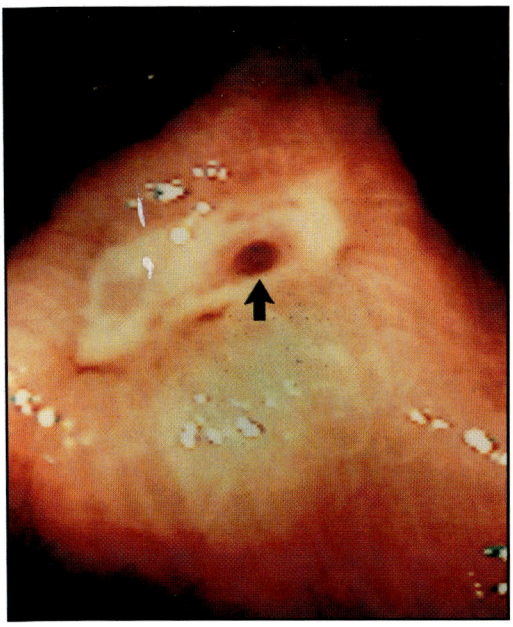

Color Plate 1–1 An atrophic vessel (*arrow*) in an ulcer crater appearing as a flat red spot. Therapy for *Helicopter pylori* was prescribed. (See Figure 1–1, page 5.)

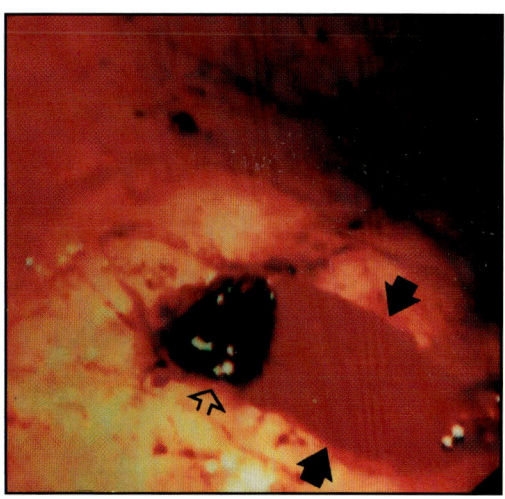

Color Plate 1–2 Active bleeding (*arrows*) from the base of a black clot (*open arrow*) obscuring an ulcer. Injection therapy was successful. (See Figure 1–2, page 6.)

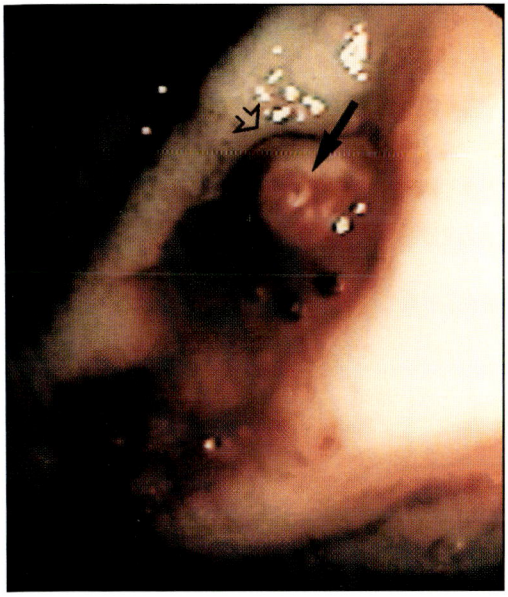

Color Plate 1–3 Visible vessel (*arrow*) with surrounding edematous folds (*open arrow*) from injection therapy. Rebleeding did not occur. (See Figure 1–3, page 6.)

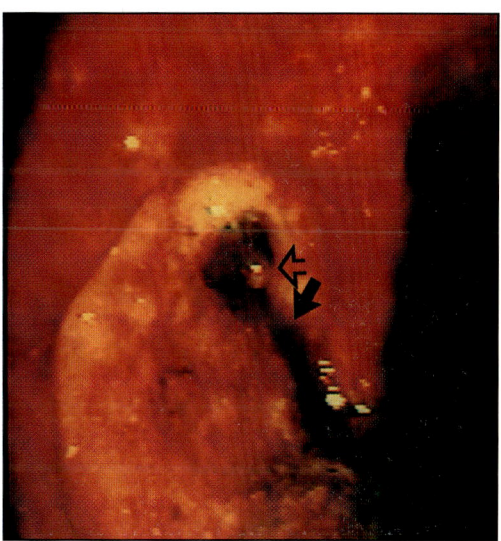

Color Plate 1–4 Minimal bleeding (*arrow*) from a pigmented protuberance (*open arrow*) in a large antral ulcer. Injection therapy halted further bleeding. (See Figure 1–4, page 6.)

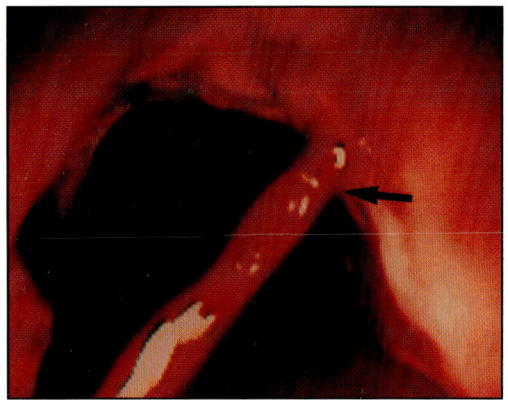

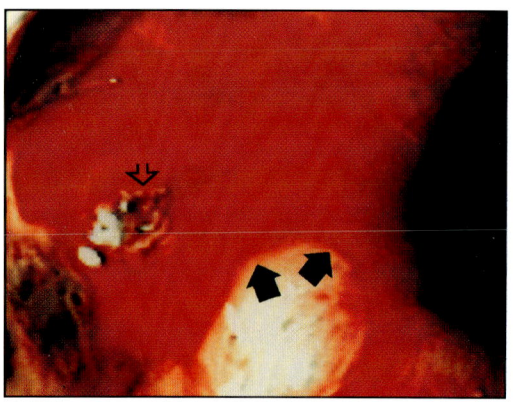

Color Plate 1–5 Active hemorrhage (*arrow*) from an esophageal varix seen only after rolling the patient to position the varix above the air-blood level. Scelerotherapy stopped the acute bleeding. (See Figure 1–5, page 7.)

Color Plate 1–7 Blood (*arrows*) oozing from a Dieulafoy's lesion (*open arrow*). Thermal coagulation was successful. (See Figure 1–7, page 9.)

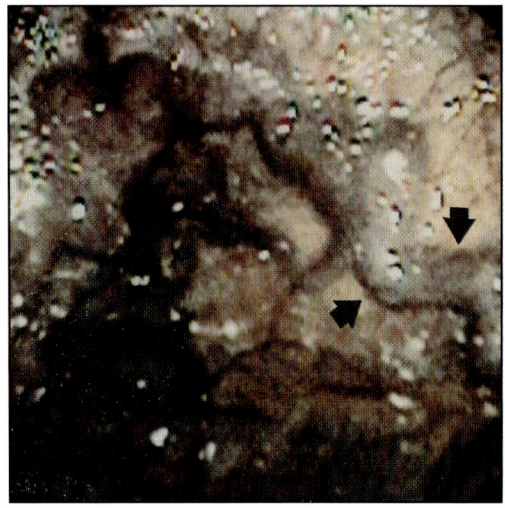

A

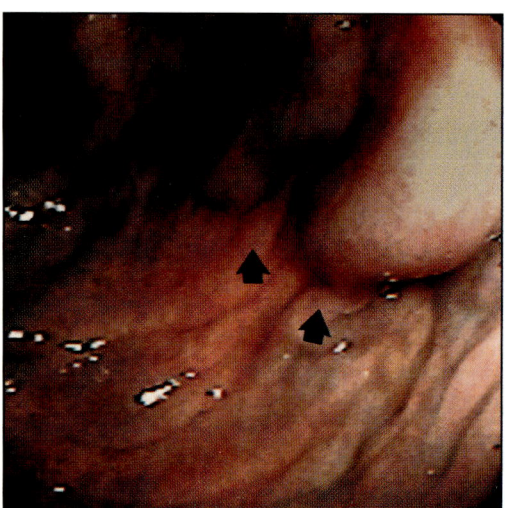

B

Color Plate 1–6 **(A)** Dark gastric varices (*arrows*) are easily recognized as veins compared with **(B)**. **(B)** Light-colored gastric varices (*arrows*) may be overlooked as prominent rugae. (See Figure 1–6, page 8.)

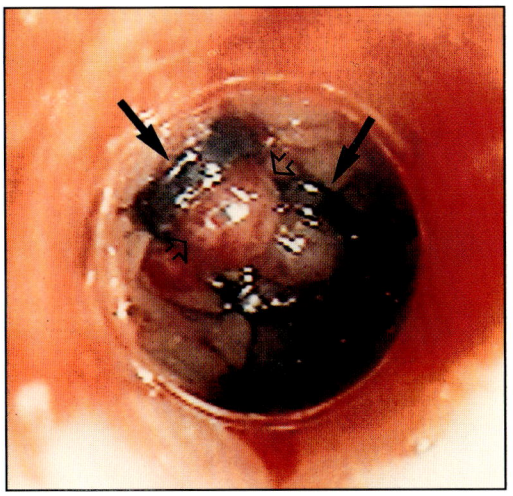

Color Plate 1–8 Endoscopic view after deploying multiple rubber bands (*arrows*) on esophageal varices (*open arrows*). (See Figure 1–8, page 11.)

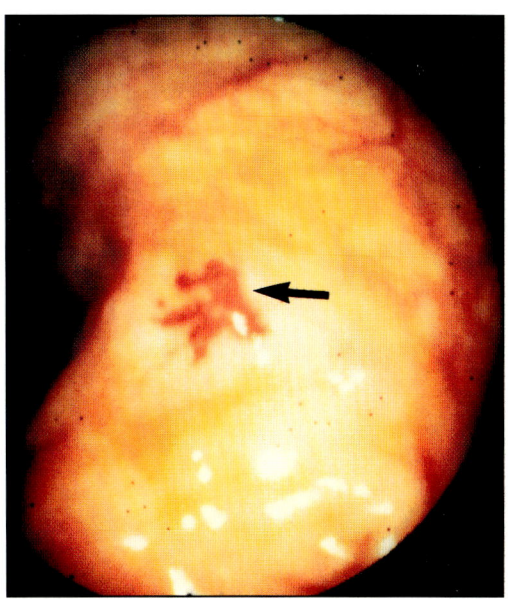

Color Plate 1–14 Prominent colonic angiodysplasia (*arrow*) in a patient with recurrent lower GI bleeding. (See Figure 1–14, page 22.)

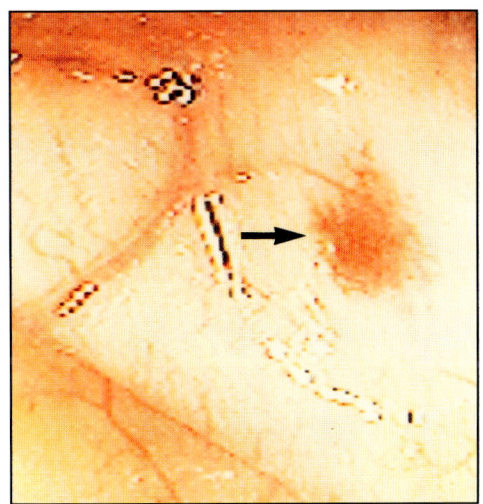
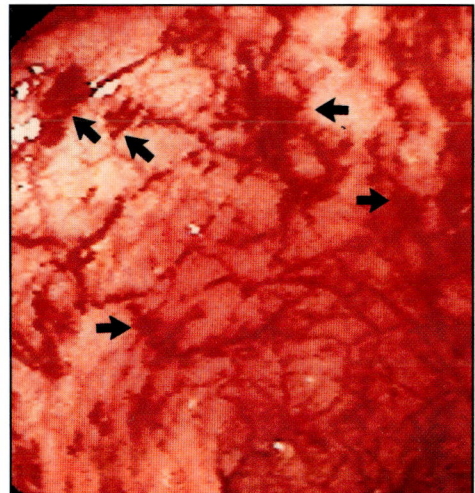

Color Plate 1–15 Colonic angiodysplasias may be **(A)** subtle (*arrow*) or **(B)** diffuse (*arrows*). (See Figure 1–15, page 23.)

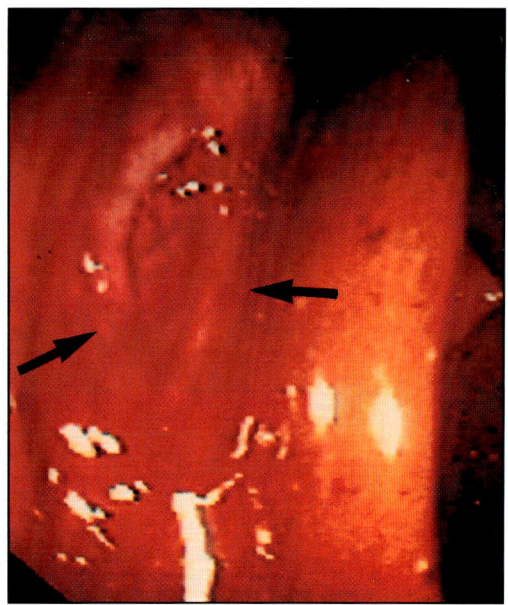

Color Plate 1–16 Inflamed diverticulum (*arrows*) with prominent vascular markings. (See Figure 1–16, page 23.)

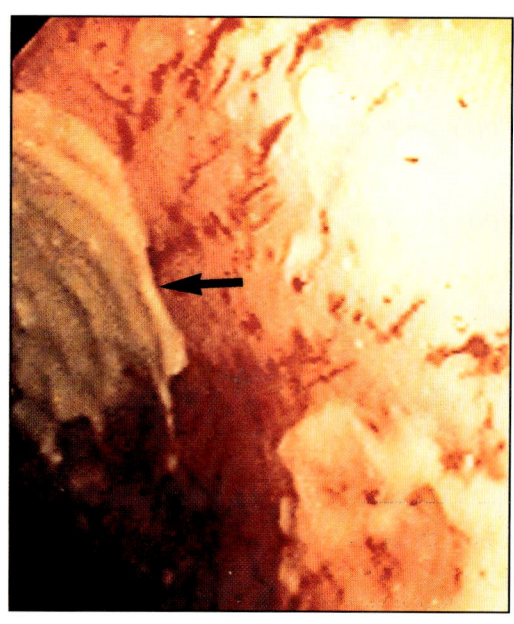

Color Plate 1–17 Plaquelike exudate (*arrow*) and punctate hemorrhage in ischemic colitis. (See Figure 1–17, page 23.)

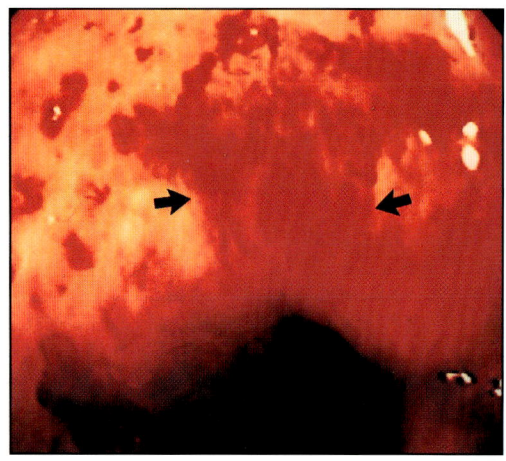

Color Plate 1–18 Diffuse blood oozing from radiation-induced colitis (*arrows*). (See Figure 1–18, page 24.)

Clearly, those individuals most likely to benefit from surgery are those who are least likely to tolerate it. Overall, indications for *emergency* operative intervention include inability to access a vessel endoscopically, a torrential bleed not amenable to endoscopic hemostasis, or an unidentified source of upper GI bleed with hemodynamic compromise. Indications for *early* operative intervention (within 24 hours, following resuscitation and endoscopic hemostasis), include age over 60 *and* any of the following: endoscopic stigmata of bleeding (active ulcer hemorrhage, visible vessel, adherent clot), a single rebleed, or loss of 4 U of blood over 24 hours.[208] Younger patients should be considered for surgery if more than 8 U of blood or colloid is required over 24 hours, or 12 U of blood or colloid is required over 48 hours, or if two episodes of rebleeding occur during the hospitalization period.[207]

Type of Operation and Surgical Technique

The choice of operation for bleeding gastric and duodenal ulcers is contingent on the physiologic status of the patient, the location of the ulcer, and the expertise and preference of the surgeon. Bleeding gastric ulcers are virulent, and the possibility of a malignancy must be excluded.[212] The gastric location confers a higher risk for recurrent bleeding [213, 214] and a greater likelihood for requiring operative intervention to obtain hemostasis than their duodenal counterparts. Gastric ulcers are also more likely to occur in older patients with more numerous comorbid health problems.[212] Early surgical intervention is therefore warranted. Traditionally, a 60% distal gastrectomy with Billroth I reconstruction, with or without vagotomy is performed. Vagotomy is performed with type 2 (with accompanying duodenal ulcers) and type 3 (pyloric channel ulcers) and is not indicated in type 1 (lesser curvature proximal to the incisura) and type 4 (esophagogastric junction) ulcers. (A vagotomy is performed in type 1 patients if drug abuse or alcohol abuse coexists in the patient.) In elderly patients who are hemodynamically compromised or have significant comorbid disease, a truncal vagotomy and pyloroplasty with suture ligation and biopsy of the ulcer is an option, although this carries a higher risk of recurrent ulceration (15%) than does gastrectomy.[215] With the advent of H_2 blockers and omeprazole, there are those who choose oversewing of the ulcer alone as an option in an especially high-risk patient.[216] The development of laparoscopic techniques shows promise for transgastric suture ligation for control of gastric ulcer bleeding. Using either a laparoscopic or combined endoscopic/laparoscopic technique, [217,218] success has been described in one human case report and in porcine trials. The results are promising, but it is recognized that this approach provides no definitive treatment of the underlying disease process. Truncal vagotomy and antrecromy with Billroth I reconstruction is the traditional procedure of choice for bleeding duodenal ulcers.[219] Other open procedures, such as truncal vagotomy and pyloroplasty and highly selective vagotomy with oversewing of the ulcer, are also op-tions but have higher rebleeding rates.[220–222] The physiologic status of the patient, history of previous ulcer disease complications, comorbid disease, and expertise of the surgeon guides the choice of operations for the acutely bleeding patient. Laparoscopic versions of truncal, selective, and highly selective vagotomy operations have evolved and are widely used in elective scenerios.[14,15,223,224] However, their use in the emergency setting is limited at this time.

LOWER GASTROINTESTINAL HEMORRHAGE

Resuscitation and Triage

Assessment and medical resuscitation of patients with lower GI bleeding is nearly identical to that with GI hemorrhage. The passing of red blood by rectum most often indicates that the bleeding site is within 60 cm of the anal verge; however, in a rapidly exsanguinating patient, a large-caliber artery bleeding into the gut lumen at any site throughout the digestive tract may be responsible. Upper endoscopy is commonly performed to exclude an upper source, followed by colonoscopic evaluation.[225,226] After or during medical resuscitation, polyethylene glycol osmotic solutions can be administered rapidly via NG tube such that adequate colonic mucosal visualization can be performed within several hours. Application of hemostatic techniques through the colonoscope can be very challenging during active bleeding due to the relatively small luminal diameter and impaired ability to see above the blood–air interface. Clinical judgment must be employed in deciding when to persist with an endoscopic exam as opposed to pursuing radiologic or surgical intervention.

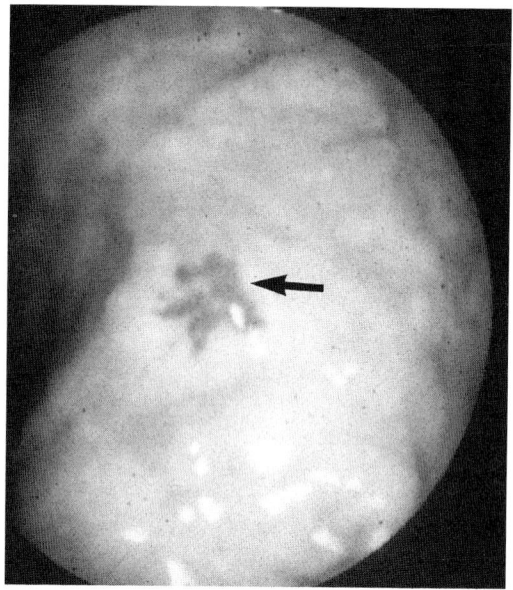

Figure 1–14 Prominent colonic angiodysplasia (*arrow*) in a patient with recurrent lower GI bleeding. (See color plate 1–14.)

Colonoscopic Findings and Interventions

As with upper GI hemorrhage, a majority of bleeding sources heal spontaneously without specific intervention. Colonoscopic exams most often serve to diagnose sites of earlier bleeding. Common colonic sources include angiodysplasias and diverticuli (Figs. 1–14, 1–15a, 15b, 1–16), with classic inflammatory bowel disease (Crohn's or ulcerative colitis) or colitis from other causes, such as ischemia (Fig. 1–17), NSAIDs, radiation (Fig. 1–18), or infection, being less common. Large ulcerating neoplasms may be the source of lower GI hemorrhage, whereas neoplasms smaller than 2 cm rarely cause overt bleeding. Anal outlet sources of bleeding include hemorrhoids, anal fissures, bleeding from mucosal tears due to foreign bodies, and distal proctitis. Bleeding in these patients is not usually massive but is nevertheless frightening to the patient because it is easily recognized as bright red blood. A history of dyschezia, or prior diagnosis of hemorrhoids with frequent small volumes of red blood, is usually indicative of anal outlet sources. Multiple nonsurgical methods for the definitive management of hemorrhoids are available and are utilized by gastroenterologists, generalists with specific training in these techniques, and surgeons. Such methods include infrared thermal cautery, rubber band ligation, bipolar electrocoagulation, and, occasionally, injection sclerosis.[227] Endoscopic treatment options for the commonly seen small-vessel angiodysplasias include thermal coagulation with heater probe, multipolar probes, or laser—all with excellent results.[158,228] In general, the energy settings are similar to upper GI tract angiodysplasia, but the tissue contact time should be shorter, especially when the lesion is in the thin-walled right colon. Monopolar techniques are inadvisable in comparison with bipolar ones due to the higher risk of perforation. A larger visible vessel or pigmented protuberance

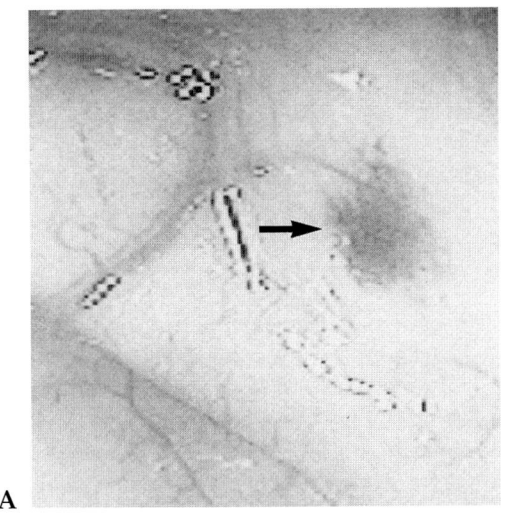
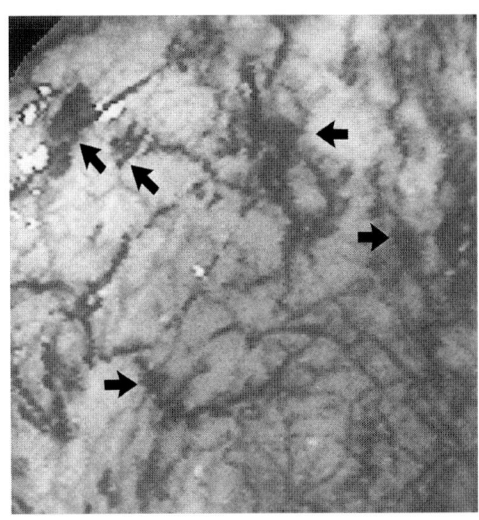

Figure 1–15 Colonic angiodysplasias may be **(A)** subtle (*arrow*) or **(B)** diffuse (*arrows*). (See color plate 1–15.)

poses a greater challenge, as the endoscopist does not have the luxury of delivering a firm, slow thermal treatment; in these circumstances, many endoscopists recommend using nonsclerosing injection agents, such as saline or diluted epinephrine. If necessary, vessel banding, clipping, sewing, or endoloop techniques can be used with efficacy and minimal risk of perforation.

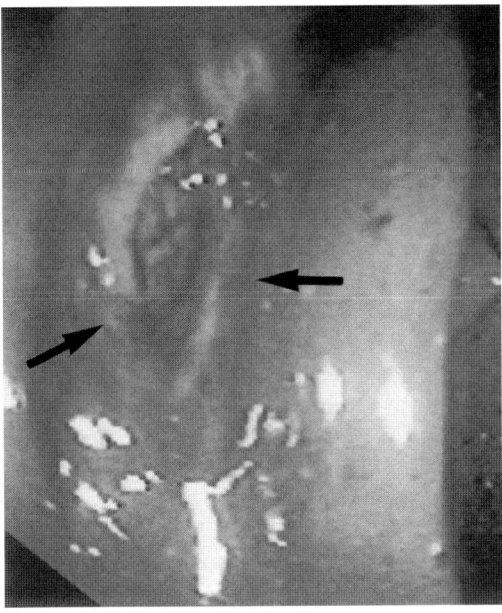

Figure 1–16 Inflamed diverticulum (*arrows*) with prominent vascular markings. (See color plate 1–16.)

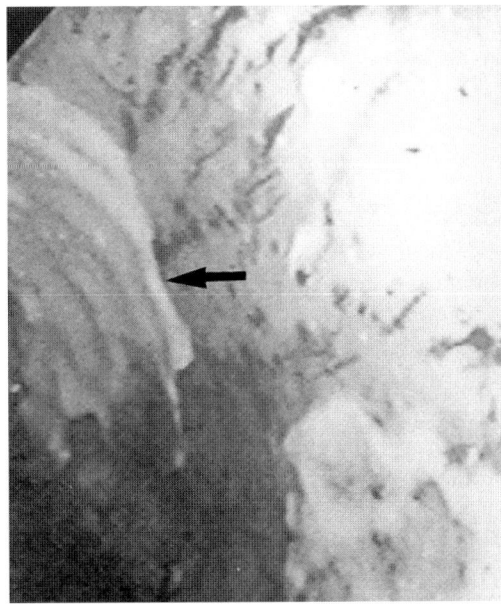

Figure 1–17 Plaquelike exudate (*arrow*) and punctate hemorrhage in ischemic colitis. (See color plate 1–17.)

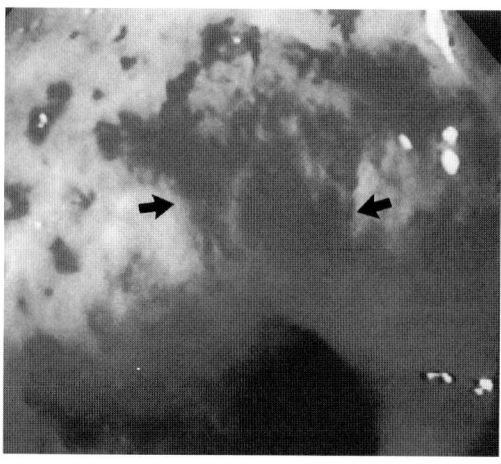

Figure 1–18 Diffuse blood oozing from radiation-induced colitis (*arrows*). (See color plate 1–18.)

Radiologic and Surgical Techniques

Patients presenting with shock who continue to remain hypotensive despite vigorous resuscitation or who continue to pass blood per rectum are not candidates for elective, prepped colonoscopy. An unprepped colonoscopic examination may be both diagnostic and therapeutic, and should be offered immediately. If an endoscopic examination cannot be done or is ineffective, angiography in the hemodynamically stable patient can pinpoint the hemorrhage. Vasoconstrictors or embolotherapy as indicated are usually successful and may preclude the need for surgery. For lower GI bleeding, ultraselect catheterizations are required in the colonic branches of the SMA and IMA for the obvious reasons that these single vessels supply a diffuse amount of bowel. This often requires placement of the microcatheter with embolization using microcoils or small Gelfoam pledgets, although PVA has also been used with success. Even with this superselectivity, as many as 10% of patients undergoing this procedure will have bowel infarction. Given the high rate of infarction, surgery is still considered the procedure of choice at this time, although embolization is finding more acceptance. In patients scheduled for elective surgery due to recurrent bleeding, preoperative angiography allows for minimal surgery tailored to the individual patient. In persistently unstable patients with lower GI hemorrhage, emergency subtotal colectomy may most expeditiously allow for hemodynamic stabilization and definitive life-saving therapy.[229]

Summary

Technological advancements over the last two decades have resulted in significant improvements in endoscopic, radiologic, and minimally invasive surgical control of a majority of patients with GI hemorrhage. A multidisciplinary approach for the resuscitation, early diagnosis, and therapy for such bleeding has resulted in reduced morbidity, reduced numbers of transfusions, reduced rebleeding rates, and reduced need for emergency surgery. That overall mortality remains around 8% is due in part to our increasingly older population, whose comorbidity contributes to lower survival. Mortality has been reduced in selected subsets of bleeding patients who undergo endoscopic control of bleeding.[13,126,134] Thorough collaboration among medical, surgical, and radiologic specialists will allow for continued progress in the care of patients with GI hemorrhage. Now that multiple efficacious therapies for acute and chronic management of GI bleeding have been developed, prospective trials should help define the optimal methods for the individual patient and specific clinical situations. End points in such trials should include comparative efficacies, morbidity and mortality, as well as cost and quality-of-life measurements.

References

1. Laine L, Peterson WL. Bleeding peptic ulcer. *N Engl J Med* 1994;331:717–728.
2. Kurath JH, Corboy ED. Current peptic ulcer time trends: an epidemiologic profile. *J Clin Gastroenterol* 1988;10:259–268.
3. Gilbert DA. Epidemiology of upper gastrointestinal bleeding. *Gastrointest Endosc* 1990;36:S8–S13.

4. Longstreth AF. Epidemiology of hospitalization for acute upper gastrointestinal hemorrhage: a population-based study. *Am J Gastroenterol* 1995;90:206–210.
5. Rockall TA, Logan RFA, Devlin HB, Northfield TC. Incidence of and mortality from acute upper gastrointestinal hemorrhage in the United Kingdom. *BMJ* 1995;331:222–226.
6. Gabriel SE, Jaakkimainen L, Bombardier C. Risks for serious gastrointestinal complications related to the use of non-steroidal anti-inflammatory drugs: a metaanalysis. *Ann Intern Med* 1991;115:787–796.
7. Garcia Rodriguez LA, Jick H. Risk of upper gastrointestinal bleeding and perforation associated with individual non-steroidal anti-inflammatory drugs. *Lancet* 1994;343:769–772.
8. Baum C, Kennedy DL, Forbes MB. Utilization of nonsteroidal anti-inflammatory drugs. *Arthritis Rheum* 1985;28:686.
9. Walsh JH, Peterson WL. The treatment of *Helicobacter pylori* infection in the management of peptic ulcer disease. *N Engl J Med* 1995;333:984–991.
10. Lewis BS. Vascular anomalies of the gastrointestinal tract. *Semin Gastrointest Dis* 1992;3:105–112.
11. Pitcher JL. Therapeutic endoscopy and bleeding ulcers: historical overview. *Gastrointest Endosc* 1990;36:S2–S7.
12. Morrissey JF. Clinical approach to diagnostic endoscopy in patients with upper gastrointestinal bleeding. *Dig Dis Sci* 1981;26:6–11.
13. Cook DJ, Guyatt GH, Salena BJ, Laine LA. Endoscopic therapy for acute nonvariceal upper gastrointestinal hemorrhage: a meta-analysis. *Gastroenterology* 1992;102:139–148.
14. Siu WT, Leong HT, Li MKW. Laparoscopic resection of bleeding gastric polyps. *Surg Endosc* 1997;11:283–284.
15. Johansson B, Hallerback B, Glise H, Johnsson E. Laparoscopic suture closure of perforated peptic ulcer. *Surg Endosc* 1996;10:656–658.
16. Gupta H, Weissleder R, Bogdanov AA Jr, Brady TJ. Experimental gastrointestinal hemorrhage: detection with contrast-enhanced MR imaging and scintigraphy. *Radiology* 1995;196:239–244.
17. Maurer AH, Rodman MS, Vitti RA, Revez G, Krevsky B. Gastrointestinal bleeding: improved localization with cine scintigraphy. *Radiology* 1992;185:187–192.
18. Athanasoulis CA. Therapeutic applications of angiography. *N Engl J Med* 1980;302:1117–1125.
19. Schmidt SP, Boskind JF, Smith DC, Catalano RD. Angiographic localization of small bowel angiodysplasia with use of platinum coils. *J Vasc Intervent Radiol* 1993;4:737–739.
20. Curtiss JR, Rice SD. Control of gastrointestinal hemorrhage in the critical care unit. *Curr Opin Crit Care* 1997;3:138–143.
21. Kollef MH, Canfield DA, Zuckerman GR. Triage considerations for patients with acute gastrointestinal hemorrhage admitted to a medical intensive care unit. *Crit Care Med* 1995;23:1048–1954.
22. Jiranek G, Kozarek R. Using endoscopy in the care of patients who have UGI bleeds. *Intern Med* 1995;238:45–56.
23. McLaughlin WD, Kolts BE, Achem SR. Nasogastric lavage compared with outcome in 101 patients seen in an emergency room for upper gastrointestinal hemorrhage (abstract). *Gastroenterology* 1987;92:1529.
24. Booker JA, Johnson M, Booder Cl, Tydd T, Mitchell R. Prognostic factors for continued or rebleeding and death from gastrointestinal hemorrhage in the elderly. *Age Ageing* 1987;16:208–214.
25. Peterson WL. Clinical risk factors. *Gastrointest Endosc* 1990;36:S14–15.
26. Bernstein DE, Jeffers L, Erhardtsen E, et al. Recombinant factor VIIa corrects prothrombin time in cirrhotic patients: a preliminary study. *Gastroenterology* 1997;113:1930–1937.
27. Choudari CP, Palmer KR. Acute gastrointestinal haemorrhage in patients treated with anticoagulant drugs. *Gut* 1995;36:483–484.
28. Lipper B, Simon D, Cerrone F. Pulmonary aspiration during emergency endoscopy in patients with upper gastrointestinal hemorrhage. *Crit Care Med* 1991;19:330–333.
29. Soriano G, Guarner C, Tomas A, et al. Norfloxacin prevents bacterial inflection in cirrhotics with gastrointestinal hemorrhage. *Gastroenterology* 1992;103:1267–1272.
30. Macleod IA, Mills PR. Factors identifying the probability of further haemorrhage after acute upper gastrointestinal haemorrhage. *Br J Surg* 1982;69:256–258.
31. Roberts LR, Kamath PS. Pathophysiology and treatment of variceal hemorrhage. *Mayo Clin Proc* 1996;71:973–983.
32. Carey WD. Pharmacologic management of

portal hypertensive upper intestinal hemorrhage. *Semin Gastrointest Dis* 1992;3:75–82.
33. Beson I, Ingrad P, Person B, et al. A comparison of octreotide combined with emergency sclerotherapy to sclerotherapy alone in the treatment of acute variceal bleeding: a randomized, double-blind, placebo controlled trial (abstract). *Gastroenterology* 1995;108:A1034.
34. Sung JY, Chung SCS, Leung VKS, et al. Octreotide as an adjuvant therapy to endoscpic variceal ligation for acute variceal hemorrhage (abstract). *Gastroenterology* 1995;108A:1034.
35. Imperiale TF, Birgisson S. Somatostatin or octreotide compared with H2 antagonists and placebo in the management of acute nonvariceal upper gastrointestinal hemorrhage: a meta-analysis. *Ann Intern Med* 1997;127:1062–1071.
36. The ltalian Multicenter Project for Propranolol in Prevention of Bleeding. Propranolol for prophylaxis of bleeding in cirrhotic patients with large varices: a multicenter study. *Hepatology* 1988;8:1–5.
37. Garden OJ, Mills PR, Birnie GG, et al. Propranolol in the prevention of recurrent variceal hemorrhage in cirrhotic patients: a controlled trial. *Gastroenterology* 1990;98:185–190.
38. Andreani T, Poupon RE, Balkau BJ, et al. Preventive therapy of first gastrointestinal bleeding in patients with cirrhosis: results of a controlled trial comparing propranolol, endoscopic sclerotherapy and placebo. *Hepatology* 1990;12:1413–1419.
39. Ideo G, Bellati G, Fesce E, et al. Nadolol can prevent first gastrointestinal bleeding in cirrhotics: a prospective randomized study. *Hepatology* 1988;8:6–9.
40. Lebrec D, Poynard T, Capron JP, et al. Nadolol for prophylaxis of gastrointestinal bleeding in patients with cirrhoiss: a randomized trial. *J Hepatol* 1988;7:118–125.
41. Jones AL, Hayes PC. Organic nitrates in portal hypertenison. *Am J Gastroenterol* 1994;89:7–14.
42. Vatner SF, Pagani M, Rutherford Y. Effect of nitrogylcerine on cardiac function and regional blood flow distribution in conscious dogs. *Am J Physiol* 1978;234:244–252.
43. Bhatal PS, Grossman HJ. Contractile fibroblasts in the pathogenesis of cirrhotic portal hypertension (abstract). *Hepatology* 1982;2:155.
44. Bhatal PS, Grossman HJ. Reduction of the increased portal vascular resistance of the isolated perfused cirrhotic rat liver by vasodilators. *J Hepatol* 1985;1:325–327.
45. Westaby D, Gimson A, Hayes PC, et al. Haemodynamic response to intravenous vasopressin and nitroglycerine in portal hypertension. *Gut* 1988;29:372–377.
46. Mols P, Hallemans R, Melot C, et al. Systemic and regional hemodynamic effects of isosorbide dinitrate in patients with liver cirrhosis and portal hypertension. *J Hepatol* 1989;8:316–324.
47. Navasca M, Chesta J, Bosch J, et al. Reduction of portal pressure by isosorbide-5-mononitrate in patients with cirrhosis. *Gastroenterology* 1989;96:1110–1118.
48. Garcia-Pagan JC, Feu F, Bosch J, et al. Propranolol compared with propranolol plus isosorbide-5-mononitrate for portal hypertension in cirrhosis: a randomized controlled study. *Ann Intern Med* 1991;114:869–873.
49. Holstege A, Palitzch KD, Scholmerich J. The role of drug treatment in variceal bleeding. *Digestion* 1994;55:1–12.
50. Jenkins SA, Baxter JN, Critchley M, et al. Randomized trial of octreotide for long term management of cirrhosis after variceal hemorrhage. *BMJ* 1997;315:1338–1341.
51. Harris RA, Kuppermann M, Richter JE. Proton pump or histamine-2 receptor antagonists for the prevention of recurrences of erosive reflux esophagitis: a cost effectiveness analysis. *Am J Gastroenterol* 1997;92: 2179–2187.
52. Ekstorm P, Carling L, Wetterhus S, et al. Prevention of peptic ulcer and dyspeptic symptoms with omeprazole in patients receiving continuous nonsteroidal anti-inflammatory drug therapy: a Nordic multicentre study. *Scand J Gastroenterol* 1996;31:753–758.
53. Cook D, Guyatt G, Marshall J, et al. A comparison of sucralfate and ranitidine for the prevention of upper gastrointestinal bleeding in patients requiring mechanical ventilation. *N Engl J Med* 1998;38:791–797.
54. Graham DY, Lew GM, Klein PD, et al. Effect of treatment of *Helicobacter pylori* infection on the long-term recurrence of gastric or duodenal ulcer. *Ann Intern Med* 1992;116:705–708.

55. Jaspersen D, Koerner T, Schorr W, et al. *Helicobacter pylori* eradication reduces the rate of rebleeding in ulcer hemorrhage. *Gastrointest Endosc* 1995;41:5–7.
56. Labenz J, Borsch G. Role of *Helicobacter pylori* eradication in the prevention of peptic ulcer bleeding relapse. *Digestion* 1994;55:19–23.
57. Graham DY, Hepps KS, Ramirez FC, et al. Treatment of *Helicobacter pylori* reduces the rate of rebleeding in peptic ulcer disease. *Scand J Gastroenterol* 1993;28:939–942.
58. Cutler AF, Goldstein JL, McDaniel R, et al. Cost effective *Hp* diagnosis after therapy. *Gut* 1996;36:A107.
59. NIH Consensus Developement Panel. *Helicobacter pylori* in peptic ulcer disease. *JAMA* 1994;272:65–69.
60. Cutler AF, Havstad S, Ma CK, et al. Accuracy of invasive and noninvasive tests to diagnose *Helicobacter pylori* infection. *Gastroenterology* 1995;109:136–141.
61. Laine L. Rolling review: upper gastrointestinal bleeding. *Aliment Pharmacol Ther* 1993;7:207–232.
62. Harris JM, DiPalma JA. Clinical significance of Mallory-Weiss tears. *Am J Gastroenterol* 1993;88:2056–2058.
63. Liberski SM, McGarrity TJ, Hartle RJ, Verano V, Reynolds D. The watermelon stomach: long-term outcome in patients treated with Nd:YAG laser therapy. *Gastrointest Endosc* 1994;40:584–587.
64. Wilcox CM, Alexander LN, Straub RF, Clark WS. A Prospective endoscopic evaluation of the causes of upper GI hemorrhage in alcoholics: a focus on alcoholic gastropathy. *Am J Gastroenterol* 1996;91:1343–1347.
65. Baettig B, Haecki W, Lammer F, Jost R. Dieulafoy's disease: endoscopic treatment and follow-up. *Gut* 1993;34:1418–1421.
66. Spechler SJ, Schimmel EM. Gastrointestinal tract bleeding of unknown origin. *Arch Intern Med* 1982;142:236–240.
67. Risti B, Marincek B, Jost R, Decurtins M, Ammon R. Hemosuccus pancreaticus as a source of obscure upper gastrointestinal bleeding: three cases and a literature review. *Am J Gastroenterol* 1995;90:1878–1880.
68. Lewis BS, Saye JD. Small bowel enteroscopy in 1988: pros and cons. *Am J Gastroenterol* 1988;83:799–802.
69. Foutch PG, Sawyer R, Sanowski RA. Push-enteroscopy for diagnosis of patients with gastrointestinal bleeding of obscure origin. *Gastrointest Endosc* 1990;36:337–341.
70. Lewis BS, Wenger JS, Wayne JD. Small bowel enteroscopy and intraoperative enteroscopy for obscure gastrointestinal bleeding. *Am J Gastroenterol* 1991;86:171–174.
71. Gostout CJ, Schroeder KW, Burton DD. Small bowel enteroscopy: an experience in gastrointestinal bleeding of unknown origin. *Gastrointest Endosc* 1991;37:5–8.
72. Nord JH. Assessing risk, managing, and monitoring bleeding peptic ulcers. *Contemp Intern Med* 1994;6:41–54.
73. Johnston JH. Endoscopic risk factors for bleeding peptic ulcer. *Gastrointest Endosc* 1990;36:S16–S20.
74. Jensen DM, Machicado G, Kovacs T, et al. Current treatment and outcome of patients with bleeding "stress ulcers." *Gastroenterology* 1988;94:A208.
75. Storey DW, Bown SG, Swain CP, Salmon PR, Kirkham JS, Northfield TC. Endoscopic prediction of recurrent bleeding in peptic ulcers. *N Engl J Med* 1981;305:915–916.
76. Yang CC, Shin JS, Lin XZ, Hsu Pl, Chen KW, Lin CY. The natural history (fading time) of stigmata of recent hemorrhage in peptic ulcer disease. *Gastrointest Endosc* 1994;40:562–566.
77. Thomopoulos KC, Nikolopoulou VN, Katsakoulis EC, et al. The effect of endoscopic injection therapy on the clinical outcome of patients with benign peptic ulcer bleeding. *Scand J Gastroenterol* 1997;32:212–216.
78. Hsu PL, Lin XZ, Chan SH. Bleeding peptic ulcer risk factors for rebleeding and sequential changes in endoscopic findings. *Gut* 1994;35:746–754.
79. Sneed ZA, Ramirez FC, Hepps KS, Cole RA, Graham DY. Prospective validation of the Baylor bleeding score for predicting the likelihood of rebleeding after endoscopic hemostasis of peptic ulcers. *Gastrointest Endosc* 1995;41:561–565.
80. NIH Consensus Developement Panel. Consensus statement on therapeutic endoscopy and bleeding ulcers. *Gastrointest Endosc* 1990;36:S62–S65.
81. Freeman ML. Endoscopic control of ulcer bleeding. *Semin Gastrointest Dis* 1992;3:65–74.
82. Crafoord C, Frenckner P. New surgical treatment of varicose veins of the esophagus. *Acta Otolaryngol* 1939;27:422–429.

83. Sarin SK, Nanda R, Sachdev G, et al. Intravariceal versus paravariceal sclerotherapy: a prospective, controlled, randomized trial. *Gut* 1987;28:657–662.
84. Terblanc J, Bornman PC, Jonker MAT, et al. Injection sclerotherapy of esophageal varices. *Semin Liver Dis* 1982;2:233–241.
85. Fujiki K, Ohkusa T, Tamura Y, Sato C. Evaluation of the effects of esophageal variscosclerosants on local vascular occlusion and systemic blood coagulation. *Gastrointest Endosc* 1995;41:212–217.
86. Saeed ZA, Ramirez FC. Endoscopic therapy of bleeding from portal hypertension. *Semin Gastrointest Dis* 1992;3:83–98.
87. The Copenhagen Esophageal Varices Sclerotherapy Project. Sclerotherapy after first variceal hemorrhage in cirrhosis: a randomized trial. *N Engl J Med* 1984;311:1594–1600.
88. Paquet KJ, Feussner H. Endoscopic sclerosis and esophageal balloon tamponade in acute hemorrhage from esophagogastric varices: a prospective controlled randomized trial. *Hepatology* 1985;5:580–583.
89. Soderlund D, Ihre T. Endoscopic sclerotherapy versus conservative management of bleeding esophageal varices. *Acta Chir Scand* 1985;151:449–456.
90. Westaby D, Hayes PC, Gimson AES, et al. Controlled clinical trial of injection sclerotherapy for active variceal bleeding. *Hepatology* 1989;9:274–277.
91. Le Moine O, Hadengue A, Moreau R, et al. Relationship between portal pressure, esophageal varices, and variceal bleeding on the basis of the stage and cause of cirrhosis. *Scand J Gastroenterol* 1997;32:731–735.
92. Westaby D, Macdougall BRD, Williams R. Improved survival following injection sclerotherapy for esophageal varices: final analysis of a controlled trial. *Hepatology* 1985;5:827–830.
93. Korula J, Balart LA, Radvan G, et al. A prospective, randomized controlled trial of chronic esophageal variceal sclerotherapy. *Hepatology* 1985;5:584–589.
94. Fleig WE, Stange EF, Hunecke R, et al. Prevention of recurrent bleeding in cirrhotics with recent variceal hemorrhage: prospective, randomized comparison of propranolol and sclerotherapy. *Hepatology* 1987;7:355–361.
95. Watanabe K, Kimura K, Matsutani S, et al. Portal hemodynamics in patients with gastric varices: a study in 230 patients with esophageal and/or gastric varices using portal vein catheterization. *Gastroenterology* 1988;95:434–440.
96. Hosking SW, Johnson AG. Gastric varices: a proposed classification leading to management. *Br J Surg* 1988;75:195–196.
97. Lee RE, Prindiville TP, Trudeau WL. Endoscopic sclerotherapy for bleeding gastric varices. *Gastointest Endosc* 1991;37:16–17.
98. Soehendra N, Nam VCh, Grimm H, et al. Endoscopic obliteration of large esophagogastric varices with bucrylate. *Endoscopy* 1986;18:25–26.
99. Ramond MJ, Valla D, Gotlib JP, et al. Endoscopic obliteration of esophagogastric varices with bucrylate. I: Clinical study in 49 patients. *Gastroenterol Clin Biol* 1986;10:575–579.
100. Rauws EAJ, Jansen PLM, Tygat GNJ. Endoscopic sclerotherapy of gastric varices with bucrylate: treatment of acute bleeding and long-term follow-up. *Gastrointest Endosc* 1991;37:242.
101. Panes J, Forne M, Marco C, et al. Controlled trial of endoscopic sclerosis in bleeding peptic ulcers. *Lancet* 1987;2:1292–1294.
102. Swain CP, Storey DW, Bown SG, et al. Nature of the bleeding vessel in recurrently bleeding gastric ulcers. *Gastroenterology* 1986;90:595–608.
103. Rutgeerts P, Broechaert H, Janssens J, et al. Comparisons of endoscopic polidocanol injection and YAG laser therapy for bleeding peptic ulcers. *Lancet* 1989;1:1164–1167.
104. Kovacs TOG, Jensen DM. Endoscopic therapies for bleeding ulcers. *Gastroviewpoint*. Rahway, NJ: Merck & Co., 1991.
105. Sugawa C. Injection therapy for the control of bleeding ulcers. *Gastrointest Endosc* 1990;36:S50–S55.
106. Rutgeerts P, Geboes K, Vantrappen G. Experimental studies of injection therapy for severe nonvariceal bleeding in dogs. *Gastroenterology* 1989;97:610–621.
107. Randall AM, Jensen DM, Hirabayashi K, Machicado GA. Controlled study of different sclerosing agents for coagulation of canine gut arteries. *Gastroenterology* 1989;90:1274–1281.
108. Tekant Y, Goh P, Alexander DJ, Isaac JR, Kum CK, Ngoi SS. Combination therapy using adrenaline and heater probe to reduce rebleeding in patients with peptic

ulcer hemorrhage: a prospective randomized trial. *Br J Surg* 1995;82:223–226.
109. *ASGE Technology Assessment Status Evaluation: Bipolar and Multipolar Accessories.* Manchester, MA: American Society of Gastrointestinal Endoscopy; February 1996.
110. Jensen DM. Heat probe for hemostasis of bleeding peptic ulcers: techniques and results of randomized controlled trials. *Gastrointest Endosc* 1990;36:S42–S49.
111. Laine L. Multipolar electrocoagulation in the treatment of peptic ulcers with nonbleeding visible vessels: a prospective controlled trial. *Ann Intern Med* 1989;110:510.
112. Laine L. Multipolar electrocoagulation in the treatment of active upper gastrointestinal hemorrhage. *N Engl J Med* 1987;316:1613.
113. O'Brien JD, Day SJ, Burnham WR. Controlled trial of small bipolar probes in bleeding peptic ulcers. *Lancet* 1986;1:464–467.
114. Laine L. Determination of the optimal technique for bipolar electrocoagulation treatment. *Gastroenterology* 1991;100:107–112.
115. Johnston JH, Jensen DM, Auth D. Experimental comparison of endoscopic yttrium-aluminum-garnet laser, electrosurgery, and heater probe for canine gut arterial coagulation: importance of compression and avoidance of erosion. *Gastroenterology* 1987;92:1101–1108.
116. Laine L. Multipolar electrocoagulation versus injection therapy in the treatment of bleeding peptic ulcers: a prospective, randomized trial. *Gastroenterology* 1989;99:1303–1306.
117. Rutgeerts P, Vantrappen G, Van Hootegem P, et al. Neodymium-YAG laser photocoagulation versus multipolar electrocoagulation for treatment of bleeding ulcers: a randomized comparison. *Gastrointest Endosc* 1987;33:199–202.
118. Goff JS. Bipolar electrocoagulation versus Nd-YAG laser photocoagulation for upper gastrointestinal bleeding lesions. *Dig Dis Sci* 1986;31:906–910.
119. Hui WM, Ng MMT, Lok ASF, Lai CL, Lau YN, Lam SK. A randomized comparative study of laser photocoagulation, heater probe, and bipolar electrocoagulation in the treatment of actively bleeding ulcers. *Gastrointest Endosc* 1991;37:299–304.
120. Sherman S, Hawes RH, Nisi R, Lehman GA. Endoscopic sphincterotomy-induced hemorrhage: treatment with multipolar electrocoagulation. *Gastrointest Endosc* 1992;38:123–126.
121. Rex DK, Blair SL, Waye JD. Colonoscopy and endoscopic therapy for delayed post-polypectomy hemorrhage. *Gastrointest Endosc* 1992;38:127–129.
122. Petrini JL, Johnson JH. Heater probe treatment for antral vascular ectasis of the antrum. *Gastrointest Endosc* 1989;35:324–328.
123. Reilly HF, Al-Kawas FH. Dieulafoy's lesion: diagnosis and management. *Dig Dis Sci* 1991;36:1702–1707.
124. Richter JM, Christensen MR, Colditz G, et al. Angiodysplasia: natural history and efficacy of therapeutic interventions. *Dig Dis Sci* 1989;34:1542–1546.
125. Rogers B. Endoscopic electrocoagulation of vascular abnormalities of the gastrointestinal tract in 51 patients. *Gastrointest Endosc* 1982;28:142–143.
126. Sacks HS, Chalmers PC, Blum AL, et al. Endoscopic hemostasis for GI bleeding: an effective therapy for bleeding peptic ulcers. *JAMA* 1990;264:494–499.
127. Nath G, Gorisch W, Keifhaber P. First laser endoscopy via a fiberoptic transmission system. *Endoscopy* 1973;5:208–213.
128. Nath G, Gorish W, Kreitmair A, Kiefhaber P. Transmission of a powerful argon beam through a fiberoptic flexible gastroscope for operative gastroscopy. *Endoscopy* 1973;5:213–215.
129. Swain CP. Laser therapy for gastrointestinal bleeding. *Gastrointest Endosc Clin North Am* 1997;7:611–639.
130. Kiefhaber P, Kiefhaber K, Huber F, Nath G. Ten years endoscopic neodymium-YAG laser coagulation in gastrointestinal hemorrhage. In: Jensen DM, Brunetaud JM, eds. *Medical Laser Endoscopy.* Dordrecht: Kluwer Academic; 1990:109–118.
131. Swain CP, Salmon PR, Kirkham JS, et al. Controlled trial of Nd:YAG laser photocoagulation in bleeding peptic ulcers. *Lancet* 1986;1:1113–1116.
132. Trudeau W, Siepler JK, Ross K, et al. Endoscopic Nd:YAG laser photocoagulation of bleeding ulcers with visible vessels (abstract). *Gastrointest Endosc* 1985;31:138.
133. Rutgeerts P, Broeckaert L, Janssens J, et al. Comparison of endoscopic polidocanol injection and YAG laser therapy for bleeding peptic ulcer. *Lancet* 1989;1:1164–1166.

134. Henry DA, White I. Endoscopic coagulation for gastrointestinal bleeding. *N Engl J Med* 1988;318:186–187.
135. Naveau S, Aubert A, Poynard T, Chaput JC. Long-term results of treatment of vascular malformations of the gastrointestinal tract by neodymium YAG laser photocoagulation. *Dig Dis Sci* 1990;35:821–826.
136. Rutgeerts P, Van Gompel F, Geboes K, et al. Long term results of treatment of vascular malformations of the gastrointestinal tract by neodymium YAG laser photocoagulation. *Gut* 1985;26:586–593.
137. Gostout CJ, Ahlquist DA, Radford CM, et al. Endoscopic laser therapy for watermelon stomach. *Gastroenterology* 1989;96:1462–1465.
138. Tsai HH, Smith J, Danesh BJ. Successful control of bleeding from gastric antral vascular ectasia (watermelon stomach) by laser photocoagulation. *Gut* 1991;32:93–94.
139. Johanns W, Jakobeit C, Luis W, et al. Non-contact argon electrocoagulation in flexible endoscopy: in vitro studies. *Z Gastroenterol* 1995;33:694–700.
140. Grund KE, Storek D, Farin G. Endoscopic argon plasma coagulation (APC): first clinical experiences in flexible endoscopy. *Endosc Surg* 1994;2:42–46.
141. Haber G, Dorais J, DuVall A, et al. Argon plasma coagulation: a new effective technique of non-contact thermal coagulation: experience in 44 cases of GI angiomata. *Gastrointest Endosc* 1996;43:293.
142. Hayashi T, Yonezawa M, Kawabara T, et al. The study of stauch clip for the treatment by endoscopy. *Gastroenterol Endosc* 1975;17:92–101.
143. Villanueva C, Balanzo J, Sabat M, et al. Injection therapy alone or with endoscopic hemoclip for bleeding peptic ulcer: preliminary results of a randomized trial. *Gastrointest Endosc* 1996;43:361.
144. Handa K, Takahashi K, Fujita R. Endoscopic hemostasis for GI bleeding. *Endoscopy* 1996;28:S66.
145. Stiegmann VG, Goff JS. Endoscopic esophageal varix ligation: preliminary clinical experience. *Gastrointest Endosc* 1988;34:113–117.
146. Stiegmann VG, Goff JS, Michaletz-Onody PA, et al. Endoscopic sclerotherapy as compared with endoscopic ligation for bleeding esophageal varices. *N Engl J Med* 1992;326:1527–1532.
147. El-Newihi H, Migicovsky B, Laine L. A prospective, randomized comparison of sclerotherapy andligation for the treatment of bleeding esophageal varices. *Gastroenterology* 1991;100:A59.
148. Lo GH, Lai KH, Cheng JS, Hwu CH, Chang CF, Chiang HT. A prospective, randomized trial of sclerotherapy versus ligation in the management of bleeding esophageal varices. *Hepatology* 1995;22:466–471.
149. Laine L, Cook D. Endoscopic ligation compared with sclerotherapy for treatment of esophageal variceal bleeding. *Ann Intern Med* 1995;123:280–287.
150. Matsui S, Inoue I, Takahei K, et al. Endoscopic band ligation for hemostasis of non-variceal upper gastrointestinal bleeding. *Endoscopy* 1996;28:S67.
151. Delis V, Balatsos V, Vamvakousis V, et al. Elastic band ligation for gastric angiodysplasias. *Endoscopy* 1996;28:S65.
152. Koutsomanis D. Endoscopic ligation in ulcer bleeding: a controlled trial. *Endoscopy* 1995;27:S18.
153. Salomon P, Berner JS, Wayne JD. Endoscopic India ink injection: a method for preparation, sterilization, and administration. *Gastrointest Endosc* 1993;39:803–805.
154. Fennerty MB, Sampliner RE, Hixson LJ, Garewal H. Effectiveness of India ink as a long-term colonic mucosal marker. *Am J Gastroenterol* 1992;87:79–81.
155. Hyman N, Waye JD. Endoscopic four quadrant tattoo for the identification of colonic lesions at surgery. *Gastrointest Endosc* 1991;37:56–58.
156. Norfleet RG. Persistence of colonic India ink tattoo (letter, comment). *Am J Gastroenterol* 1992;87:1228.
157. Willis JR, Clouse RE. Medical management of GI vascular ectasia disorders. *Contemp Intern Med* 1996;8:21–33.
158. Gupta N, Longo WE, Vernava AM. Angiodysplasia of the lower gastrointestinal tract: an entity readily diagnosed by colonoscopy and primarily managed nonoperatively. *Dis Colon Rectum* 1995;38:979–982.
159. Bentley DE, Richardson JD. The role of tagged red blood cell imaging in the localization of gastrointestinal bleeding. *Arch Surg* 1991;126:821–824.
160. Greenfield AJ, Waltman AC, Athanasoulis

CA. Vasopressin in control of gastrointestinal hemorrhage: complications of selective intraarterial versus systemic infusion. *Gastroenterology* 1979;76:1114.
161. Baum S. Angiography and the gastrointestinal bleeder. *Radiology* 1982 (May); 143:569–572.
162. Malden ES, Hicks ME, Royal HD, Aliperti G, Allen BT, Picus D. Recurrent gastrointestinal bleeding: use of thrombolysis with anticoagulation in diagnosis. *Radiology* 1998; 207(1):147–151.
163. Glickerman DJ, Kowdley KV, Rosch J. Urokinase in gastrointestinal tract bleeding. *Radiology* 1988;168(2):375–376.
164. Trojanowski JQ, Harrist TJ, Athansoulis CA. Hepatic and splenic infarctions: complications of therapeutic transcatheter embolization. *Am J Surg* 1980;139:272.
165. Kelemouridis V, Athanasoulis CA, Waltman AC. Gastric bleeding sites: an angiographic study. *Radiology* 1983;149:643–648.
166. Clark RA. Intraarterial vasopressin infusion for treatment of Mallory-Weiss tears of the esophagogastric junction. *Am J Roentgenol* 1979;133:449–451.
167. Eckstein MR, Kelemouridis V, Athanasoulis CA, Waltman AC, Feldman L, Breda A. Gastric bleeding: therapy with intraarterial vasopressin and transcatheter embolization. *Radiology* 1984;152: 643–646.
168. Gomes AS, Lois JF, McCoy RD. Angiographic treatment of gastrointestinal hemorrhage: comparison of vasopressin infusion and embolization. *Am J Roentgenol* 1986;146:1031–1037.
169. Hamlin JA, Petersen B, Keller FS, Rosch J. Angiographic evaluation and management of nonvariceal upper gastrointestinal bleeding. *Gastrointest Endosc Clin North Am* 1997;7:703–716.
170. Sanblom P. *Hemobilia (Biliary Tract Hemorrhage): History, Pathology, Diagnosis, Treatment*. Springfield, IL: Charles C Thomas, 1972.
171. Rosch J, Putnam JA, Keller FS. Diagnosis and management of hemobilia. *Semin Intervent Radiol* 1988;5:49–60.
172. Sanyal AJ, Freedman AM, Luketic VA, et al. Transjugular intrahepatic portosystemic shunts for patients with active variceal hemorrhage unresponsive to sclerotherapy. *Gastroenterology* 1996;111:138–146.
173. Stanley AJ, Redhead DN, Hayes PC. Review article: update on the role of transjugular intrahepatic portosystemic stent-shunt (TIPSS) in the management of complications of portal hypertension. *Aliment Pharmacol Ther* 1997;11:261–272.
174. Shiffman ML, Jeffers L, Hoofnagle JH, Tralka TS. The role of transjugular intrahepatic portosystemic shunt for treatment of portal hypertension and its complications: a conference sponsored by the National Digestive Diseases Advisory Board. *Hepatology* 1995;22:1591–1597.
175. LaBerge JM, Ring EJ, Gordon RL, et al. Creation of transjugular intrahepatic portosystemic shunts with the Wallstent endoprosthesis: results in 100 patients. *Radiology* 1993;187:413–420.
176. Cabrera J, Maynar M, Granados R, et al. Transjugular intrahepatic portosystemic shunt versus sclerotherapy in the elective treatment of variceal hemorrhage. *Gastroenterology* 1996;110:832–839.
177. Rossle M, Deibert P, Haag K, et al. Randomized trial of transjugular-intrahepatic-portosystemic shunt versus endoscopy plus propranolol for prevention of variceal rebleeding. *Lancet* 1997;349:1043–1049.
178. Cello JP, Ring EJ, Olcott EW, et al. Endoscopic sclerotherapy compared with percutaneous transjugular intrahepatic portosystemic shunt after initial sclerotherapy in patients with acute variceal hemorrhage: a randomized, controlled trial. *Ann Intern Med* 1997;126:858–865.
179. Sanyal AJ, Freedman AM, Luketic VA, et al. Transjugular intrahepatic portosystemic shunts compared with endoscopic sclerotherapy for the prevention of recurrent variceal hemorrhage: a randomized, controlled trial. *Ann Intern Med* 1997;126: 849–857.
180. Conn HO. Hemolysis after transjugular intrahepatic portosystemic shunting: the naked stent syndrome. *Hepatology* 1996;23: 177–181.
181. Sanyal AJ, Freedman AM, Purdum PP, Shiffman ML, Luketic VA. The hematological consequences of transjugular intrahepatic portosystemic shunts. *Hepatology* 1996;23:32–39.
182. Stanley AJ, Jalan R, Forrest EH, Redhead DN, Hayes PC. Longterm follow up of transjugular intrahepatic portosystemic stent shunt (TIPSS) for the treatment of portal

hypertension: results in 130 patients. *Gut* 1996;39:479–485.
183. Sauer P, Theilmann L, Herrmann S, et al. Phenprocoumon for prevention of shunt occlusion after transjugular intrahepatic portosystemic stent shunt: a randomized trial. *Hepatology* 1996;24:1433–1436.
184. Jalan R, Harrison DJ, Redhead DN, Hayes PC. Transjugular intrahepatic portosystemic stent-shunt (TIPSS) and the role of biliary venous fistulae. *J Hepatol* 1996;24: 169–176.
185. Van Der Linden P, Le Moine O, Ghysels M, Ortinez M, Deviere J. Pulmonary hypertension after transjugular intrahepatic portosystemic shunt: effects on right ventricular function. *Hepatology* 1996;23:982–987.
186. Azoulay D, Castaing D, Dennison A, et al. Transjugular intrahepatic portosystemic shunt worsens the hyperdynamic circulatory state of the cirrhotic patient: preliminary report of a prospective study. *Hepatology* 1994;19:129–132.
187. Quiroga J, Sangro B, Nunez M, et al. Transjugular intrahepatic portal-systemic shunt in the treatment of refractory ascites: effect on clinical, renal, humoral, and hemodynamic parameters. *Hepatology* 1995; 21: 986–994.
188. Wong F, Sniderman K, Liu P, et al. Transjugular intrahepatic portosystemic stent shunt: effects on hemodynamics and sodium homeostasis in cirrhosis and refractory ascites. *Ann Intern Med* 1995;122: 816–822.
189. Wong F, Sniderman K, Liu P, Blendis L. The mechanism of the initial natriuresis after transjugular intrahepatic portosystemic shunt. *Gastroenterology* 1997;112:899–907.
190. Brensing KA, Textor J, Strunk H, et al. Transjugular intrahepatic portosystemic stent-shunt for hepatorenal syndrome. *Lancet* 1997;349:697–698.
191. Gordon FD, Anastopoulos HT, Crenshaw W, et al. The successful treatment of symptomatic, refractory hepatic hydrothorax with transjugular intrahepatic portosystemic shunt. *Hepatology* 1997;25:1366–1369.
192. Strauss RM, Martin LG, Kaufman SL, Boyer TD. Transjugular intrahepatic portal systemic shunt for the management of symptomatic cirrhotic hydrothorax. *Am J Gastroenterol* 1994;89:1520–1522.
193. Ochs A, Rossle M, Haag K, et al. The transjugular intrahepatic portosystemic stent-shunt procedure for refractory ascites. *N Engl J Med* 1995;332:1192–1197.
194. Lebrec D, Giuily N, Hadengue A, et al. Transjugular intrahepatic portosystemic shunts: comparison with paracentesis in patients with cirrhosis and refractory ascites: a randomized trial. *J Hepatol* 1996;25:135–144.
195. Martinet JP, Fenyves D, Legault L, et al. Treatment of refractory ascites using transjugular intrahepatic portosystemic shunt (TIPS): a caution. *Dig Dis Sci* 1997;42: 161–166.
196. Ng EKW, Chung SCS, Lau JTF, et al. Risk of further ulcer complications after an episode of peptic ulcer bleeding. *Br J Surg* 1996;83:840–844.
197. Jensen DM, Cheng S, Kovacs TOG, et al. A controlled study of ranitidine for the prevention of recurrent hemorrhage from duodenal ulcer. *N Engl J Med* 1994;330: 382–386.
198. Park KGM, Steele RJ, Mollison J, Crofts TJ. Prediction of recurrent bleeding after endoscopic haemostasis in non-variceal upper gastrointestinal haemorrhage. *Br J Surg* 1994; 81: 1465–1468.
199. Brullet E, Donoso L, et al. Factors predicting failure of endoscopic therapy in bleeding duodenal ulcer. *Gastroint Endosc* 1996; 43(2): part 1.
200. Choudari CP, Palmer KR. Failures of endoscopic therapy for bleeding peptic ulcer: an analysis of risk factors. *Am J Gastroenterol* 1994;89(11).
201. Hsu P-I, Chen K-W. Bleeding peptic ulcer-risk factors for rebleeding and sequential changes in endoscopic findings. *Gut* 1994;35:746–749.
202. Hunt PS. The surgical management of bleeding chronic peptic ulcer: a 10 year prospective study. *World J Surg* 1987;11: 289–294.
203. Northfield TC. Factors predisposing to recurrent haemorrhage after acute gastrointestinal bleeding. *BMJ* 1971;1:26–28.
204. Schriller KFR, Truelove SC, Gwyn Williams D. Haematemesis and melaena, with special reference to factors influencing the outcome. *Br Med J* 1970;2:7–14.
205. Benders JS, Bouwman DL, Weaver DW. Bleeding gastroduodenal ulcers: improved

outcome from a unified surgical approach. *Am Surg* 1994;60:313–315.
206. Mueller X, Rothenbuehler JM, Amert A, et al. Outcome of peptic ulcer hemorrhage treated according to a defined approach. *World J Surg* 1994;18:406–409.
207. Wheatley KE, Snyman JH, Bearley S, et al. Mortality in patients with bleeding peptic ulcer when those aged 60 or over are operated on early. *BMJ* 1990;301:272.
208. Morris DL, Hawker PC, Brearley S, et al. Optimal timing of operation for bleeding peptic ulcer: prospective randomized trial. *BMJ* 1984;288:1277–1280.
209. Chung SCS. Surgery and gastrointestinal bleeding. *Gastrointest Endosc Clin North Am* 1997;7:687–701.
210. Lau JYW, Sung JJY, Lam Y, et al. Endoscopic retreatment compared with surgery in patients with recurrent bleeding after initial endosocpic control of bleeding ulcers. *N Engl J Med* 1999;340(10):751–756.
211. Qvist P, Arnesen KE, Jacobsen CD, Rosseland AR. Endoscopic treatment and restrictive surgical policy in the management of peptic ulcer bleeding: five years experience in a central hospital. *Scand J Gastroenterol* 1994;29(6):569–576.
212. Cochran TA. Bleeding peptic ulcer: surgical therapy. *Gastroenterol Clin North Am* 1993;22(4):751–778.
213. Brearly S, Hawker PC, Morris DL, Dykes PW, Keaghley MR. Selection of patients for surgery following peptic ulcer hemorrhage. *Br J Surg* 1987;4:893–896.
214. Hunt PS. Bleeding gastroduodenal ulcers: selection of patients for surgery. *World J Surg* 1987;11:289–294.
215. Herrington JL Jr., Davidson JBA. Bleeding gastroduodenal ulcers: choice of operations. *World J Surg* 1987;11:304–314.
216. Rogers PN, Murray WR, Shaw R, Brar S. Surgical management of bleeding gastric ulceration. *Br J Surg* 1988; 75:16–17.
217. Kitano S, Kawanaka H, Tomikawa M, Hirabayashi H, Hashizume M, Sugimachi K. Bleeding form gastric ulcer halted by laparoscopic suture ligation. *Surg Endosc* 1994;8(5):405–407.
218. Potvin M, Gagner M, Pomp A. Laparoscopic transgastric suturing for bleeding peptic ulcers. *Surg Endosc* 1996;10(4):400–402.
219. Dudnick R. Management of bleeding ulcers. *Med Clin North Am* 1991;75(4):947–965.
220. Millat B, Jay J-M, Valleur P, et al. Emergency surgical treatment for bleeding duodenal ulcer: oversewing plus vagotomy versus gastric resection, a controlled randomized trial. *World J Surg* 1993;17:568–574.
221. Poxon VA, Keighley MRB, Dykes PW, et al. Comparison of minimal and conventional surgery in patients with bleeding peptic ulcer: a multicentre trial. *Br J Surg* 1991;78:1344–1345.
222. Johnston D. Division and repair of the sphincteric mechanism at the gastric outlet in emergent operations for bleeding peptic ulcer: a new technique for use in combination with suture ligation and the bleeding point at highly selective vagotomy. *Ann Surg* 1977;186:723–729.
223. Katkhouda N, Mouiel J. A new technique of surgical treatment of chronic duodenal ulcer without laparotomy by videocoelioscopy. *Am J Surg* 1991;161:361–364.
224. Casas A, Gadacz TR. Laparoscopic management of peptic ulcer disease. *Surg Clin North Am* 1996;76(3):515–522.
225. Bono MJ. Lower gastrointestinal tract bleeding. *Emerg Med Clin North Am* 1996;14:547–556.
226. Kouraklis G, Mislakos E, Karatzas G, Gogas J, Skalkeas G. Diagnostic approach and management of active lower gastrointestinal hemorrhage. *Int Surg* 1995;80:138–140.
227. Pfenninger JL. Nonsurgical treatment options for internal hemorrhoids. *Am Fam Phys* 1995;52:821–834.
228. Bonheim NA. Endoscopic therapy of bleeding gastrointestinal hemangiomas and angiodysplasia. *Am J Gastroenterol* 1985;80:727–729.
229. Drapanas T, Pennington DG, Kappelman M, Lindsey EJ. Emergency subtotal colectomy: preferred approach to management of massively bleeding diverticular disease. *Ann Surg* 1973;177:519–526.

Chapter 2

Gastrointestinal Stenting: Indications and Techniques

Mark G. Cowling
Andreas Adam

Self-expanding metallic stents are used frequently in many organs, including biliary tract, tracheobronchial tree, and vascular system. In the gastrointestinal (GI) tract they are most often employed in the esophagus, although gastric antral/pyloric, duodenal, and rectosigmoid stenting have also been described. In this chapter, we shall outline the indications for stent insertion at various sites in the GI tract, techniques employed, results, as well as complications and their management. We will also briefly mention the use of tissue adhesives as an alternative approach to dealing with esophageal fistulae and leaks into the respiratory tract.

ESOPHAGEAL STENTING

The majority of esophageal stents in our practice are inserted for palliation of malignant dysphagia caused by esophageal carcinoma (Fig. 2–1) or by extrinsic compression from malignant lymph nodes or masses. Stents may also be used to palliate tumor recurrence at surgical anastomoses, and we have occasionally had to resort to the use of stents in the treatment of benign strictures that responded poorly to balloon dilatation. Tracheoesophageal fistulae and esophageal leaks can also be successfully treated with covered stents.

Esophageal carcinoma is a relatively common disease with a poor prognosis, accounting for 3500 deaths per year in the United Kingdom[1] and ranking as the seventh most common malignancy worldwide.[2] At the time of presentation, 75% of patients have disease spread to lymph nodes,[3] and approximately 50 to 60% of patients are not suitable for attempted curative surgical resection. Available palliative treatments include surgery, radiotherapy, chemotherapy, use of rigid plastic tubes, laser therapy, and the use of self-expanding metallic esophageal stents.

Stent Types

A variety of covered and uncovered stents are available. The three most commonly used are the Wallstent (Schneider AG, Zurich, Switzerland), the Strecker stent (Boston Scientific Corporation, Watertown, MA, USA), and the Gianturco stent (William Cook Europe, Bjaeverskov, Denmark).

The Wallstent is made from a stainless steel alloy tubular mesh available in its covered form in two sizes for use in the esophagus: 20 mm diameter and 110 mm length, or 25 mm diameter and 105 mm length. The most commonly used Wallstents have a polyurethane coating on the outer surface, except for 15 mm at each end, though an uncovered esophageal Wallstent is also available. The delivery system consists of three coaxially arranged shafts in which the compressed stent is mounted. This arrangement allows partial release of the distal half of the stent, with the facility

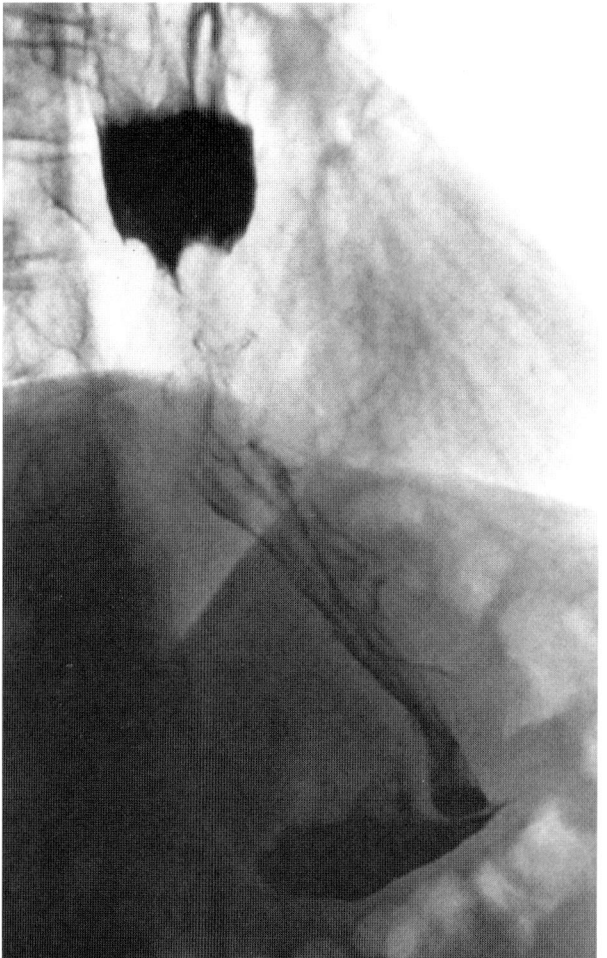
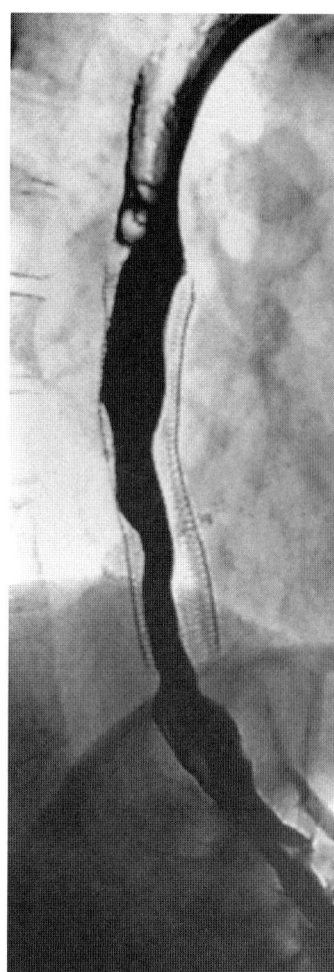

Figure 2–1 **(A)** Contrast esophagogram demonstrating a tight stricture at the esophagogastric junction due to an adenocarcinoma. **(B)** After insertion of a Strecker stent, barium is seen to flow freely into the stomach. This patient experienced excellent palliation of dysphagia and was able to tolerate a normal diet.

to reposition it prior to full deployment, either by recovering the stent and moving it to a more distal position, or by leaving the distal end partially deployed and gradually withdrawing the delivery system to the desired point. Wallstents with an outer polyurethane covering have been shown to have a high migration rate, especially when used to treat low esophageal strictures where the stent has to be placed across the gastroesophageal junction. They are now being superseded by a new design, which is conical and has an inner polyurethane covering, allowing the mesh of the stent to come directly into contact with the esophageal mucosa, thus increasing friction.

The uncovered Strecker stent is made from knitted nitinol, an alloy with thermal memory characteristics. It is available in a single diameter (18 mm), with lengths of 7, 10, or 15 cm. Until recently, the stent has been compressed onto the delivery system encased in gelatin, which dissolves after retraction of the outer sheath, thus allowing the stent to deploy. It is important to leave the delivery system in situ for several minutes to allow dissolution of the gelatin to occur because any early attempt at removal of the delivery system prior to adequate stent expansion is likely to lead to displacement or buckling of the endoprosthesis. This system can create difficulties when sedation has been less than adequate and the patient is restless. Recently, a covered Strecker stent became available; this one is compressed onto the shaft of the delivery system by a thick woven silk suture. When the stent has been correctly positioned, the suture is pulled, thus unraveling, and the stent is progressively released. This permits quicker deployment and gives the capacity for some adjustment to stent position after initial partial distal release. The Strecker esophageal stent provides a lower degree of outward radial force than the other stents that are available.

The Gianturco stent is composed of 2-cm-long basic units made from 0.018-in. stainless steel wire bent in a zig-zag pattern. The units are sutured together to form prostheses ranging in length from 4.5 to 18 cm. Various modifications on this basic design are available, but all are covered with polyurethane and have barbs to prevent migration.

The choice of stent depends to some extent on personal preference, though, as will be described later, the different stents available have certain advantages and disadvantages that have been demonstrated in a number of studies.

Technique of Insertion

An initial contrast swallow is performed to delineate the site and length of the lesion to be treated (Fig. 2–2A). At this point the size of stent required and/or the necessity for the use of more than one stent can be decided. After obtaining informed consent, the patient lies on the fluoroscopic table in the left lateral position. Xylocaine spray is applied to the pharynx, and the patient is sedated with an intravenous agent such as midazolam. Suitable catheters and guide wires are used to cross the stricture (Fig. 2–2B). In very tight strictures or in cases of esophageal occlusion, hydrophilic guide wires are valuable. The catheter and guide wire are manipulated into the duodenum to provide as stable a position as possible, and the guide wire is exchanged for an Amplatz stiff exchange wire. A 15-mm-diameter balloon is used to predilate the stricture prior to stent deployment (Fig. 2–2C). After dilatation the stent is deployed according to the technique for that particular system (Fig. 2–2D). Due to its weaker radial force the Strecker stent often requires additonal balloon dilatation. We aim to deploy the stent with approximately 60% of its length above the middle of the stricture in an effort to minimize the incidence of distal stent migration. Long strictures may require the use of more than one overlapping stent.

Immediately after the procedure, nonionic contrast medium is introduced into the esophagus via the catheter to expose procedural complications, especially esophageal perforation, and to confirm stent patency. Patients remain in hospital overnight, and once they have recovered from the effects of the sedation, they are allowed to take small volumes of clear fluids orally. The following day another contrast esophagogram is obtained to determine if further intervention is required. For example, a stent may show persistent narrowing, requiring balloon dilatation, or there may have been migration, requiring the insertion of an additional stent coaxially within the first endoprosthesis and overlapping with it to prevent further slippage. If the esophagogram shows good stent position and function, then patients are allowed a normal diet. They are advised to cut their food into small pieces, to chew it thoroughly, and to have carbonated beverages after each meal to clear the stent of any food debris.

Any patient in whom a stent has been placed across the gastroesophageal junction will eventually experience reflux of gastric contents. The symptoms are controlled by the administration of omeprazole (a suppressor of gastric acid secretion), which is routinely started after the procedure.

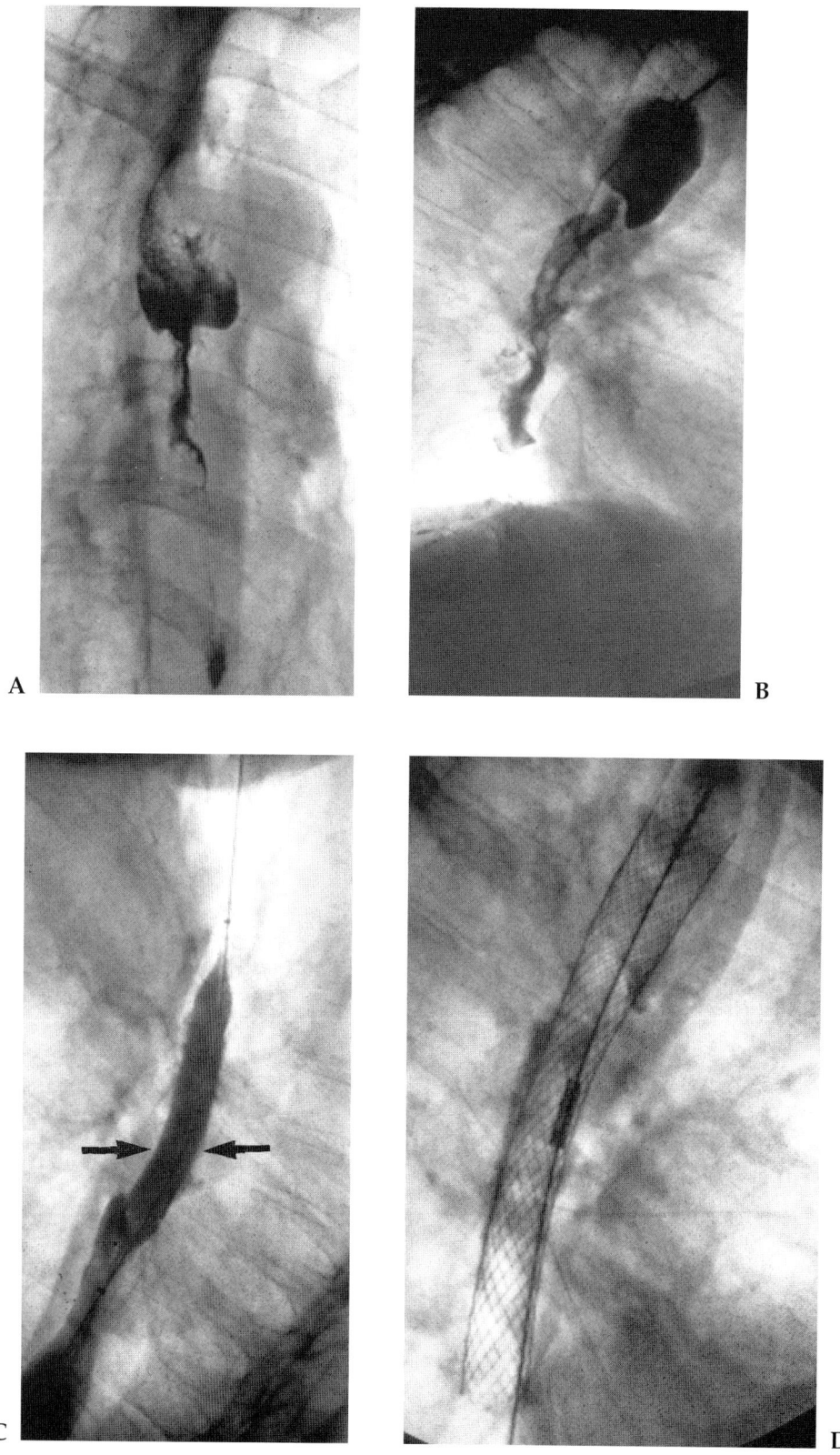

Table 2–1 Dysphagia Scoring System

Dysphagia Score	Degree of Dysphagia
0	No dysphagia
1	Able to swallow semisolid food only
2	Able to swallow liquids only
3	Difficulty in swallowing liquids and saliva
4	Complete dysphagia

Results of Esophageal Stenting in Malignant Disease

The degree of dysphagia can be assessed by the use of a dysphagia score, where 0 is equivalent to no dysphagia and 4 indicates total dysphagia (Table 2–1). The overall results of six recently published series are summarized in Table 2–2.[4–10] All of the procedures were conducted without general anesthesia and were technically successful, though there were some instances of initial stent misplacement requiring deployment of a second device. Improvement in the dysphagia score can be expected in 83 to 100% of patients when they are assessed 24 hours after the procedure.[4–9] Our experience at St. George's Hospital, for example, showed improvement from a mean dysphagia score of 2.6 prior to stenting to 0.5 after stent placement.[9]

The difference in the stent designs means that they are susceptible to different types of complications. Thus, the Strecker stent with its weaker radial force often requires additional postdeployment balloon dilatation. In addition, the Strecker stent is too weak to be used in cases of malignant dysphagia due to extrinsic compression. Its use in this situation has been reported to be associated with recurrence of dysphagia due to stent collapse.[9] Therefore, the use of the stronger Wallstent is recommended in cases of dysphagia due to extrinsic compression. Uncovered Strecker stents are prone to tumor ingrowth (20 to 30%). The lack of an outer covering probably also accounts for the absence of migration with this type of stent.

Both Wallstents and Gianturco stents are associated with an incidence of 1.5 to 15% of delayed upper GI hemorrhage. In the Guy's Hospital experience, autopsies were performed on the patients who died from hemorrhage, and no causal relationship between the stent and bleeding could be found. Other complications include severe pain, aspiration pneumonia, fistula formation (Fig. 2–3), and stent migration. The latter complication occurs in 30% of covered Wall stents and 10 to 15% of Gianturco stents. Covered stents are particularly liable to migrate when positioned at the gastroesophageal junction, with a free end lying in the stomach. The essential factor appears to be the stent covering, which reduces the friction between the esophageal wall and the stent. Wallstents rely on the uncovered portion at either end to prevent migration, and if one end lies free in the stomach this mechanism is compromised. Tumor ingrowth is seen in up to 2% of patients treated with covered stents (Fig. 2–4). In cases of complete and symptomatic stent migration, the stent can be removed by surgical gastrotomy. In cases of partial migration, the covered stent can be stabilized by the placement of a second uncovered coaxial stent through its proximal end. Because of the propensity of covered stents placed over the gastroesophageal junction to migrate, we now elect to

Figure 2–2 (A) Contrast esophagogram showing a long esophageal stricture caused by squamous carcinoma. (B) A catheter has been inserted into the esophagus part way along the stricture and contrast fluid injected to delineate the lesion. (C) The stricture is predilated with a 15-mm-diameter esophageal balloon (*arrows*). (D) Appearance immediately after deployment of a 20-mm-diameter Wallstent.

Table 2–2 Review of Six Series of Expandable Metallic Stents and Their Complications

Authors	Type of Stent	No. of Patients	Perf. (%)	Hemorr. (%)	Migration (%)	Tumor over (%)	Tumor in (%)
Cwiekiel et al[4]	Strecker	40	2.5	5.0	2.5	2.5	20
May et al[7]	Strecker	30	3.0	0	0	30.0	—
Miyayama et al[6]	Gianturco	27	0	15.0	15.0	15.0	0
Saxon et al[5]	Gianturco	52	2.0	6.0	10.0	v8.0	0
Song et al[8]	Gianturco	119	0	3.0	10.0	8.0	0
Cowling et al[9]	Streck+Wall	70	0	2.9	2.9	—	8.6

deploy uncovered stents proximally at this site, although as new Wallstent designs become available our practice may change. For example, early experience suggests that a conical design may reduce the incidence of distal migration, though in a pilot study we found that proximal migration occurred in 2 of 10 conical stents.

Recurrence of dysphagia secondary to tumor ingrowth or overgrowth can be successfully managed either with endoscopic laser therapy or by placement of additional stents. Food bolus impaction is easily cleared endoscopically.

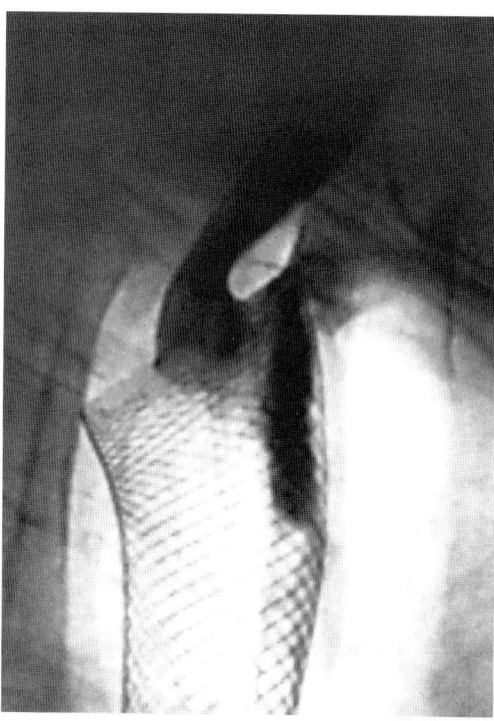

Figure 2–3 Tracheoesophageal fistula related to the upper end of a Wallstent that had been in situ for 3 months. There was no evidence that this was due to tumor, and it is presumed to have been caused by pressure necrosis.

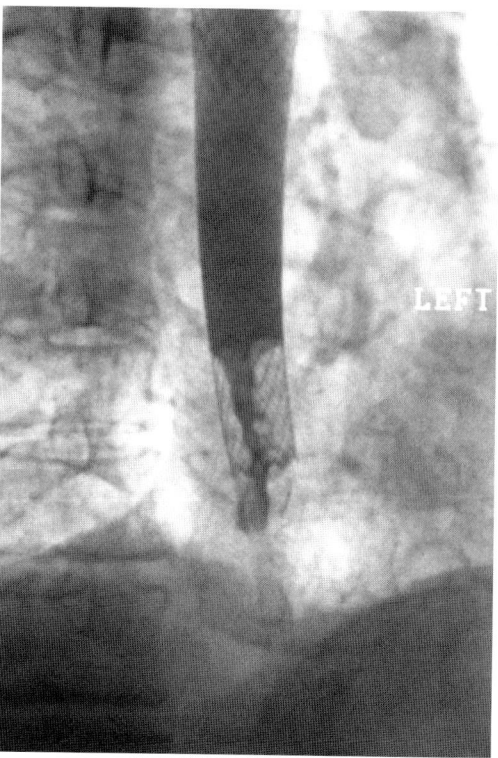

Figure 2–4 Patient had developed recurrent dysphagia 9 weeks after insertion of a covered Wall stent. Contrast esophagography demonstrated tumor ingrowth into the uncovered section at the lower end of the stent. The covered portion of the stent remains unaffected.

Comparison with Other Techniques

Conventional palliative therapy for advanced esophageal carcinoma includes surgery, radiotherapy, and chemotherapy. Palliative surgical resection is highly invasive and is associated with a high operative mortality and morbidity.[11–14] External-beam radiotherapy improves dysphagia in around 50% of patients, but at the expense of fibrotic stricutre formation in approximately 30%.[15–19] Intracavitary brachytherapy, either alone or in combination with external-beam radiotherapy, gives better results[20–22] but has the major drawback of causing esophagitis in up to 80% of patients.[22,23] Combined chemotherapy and radiotherapy also produce improved results, but with greater morbidity.[24–28]

Rigid plastic tubes, usually inserted under general anesthesia, have declined in popularity in many centers. The overal complication rate has been reported to be as high as 36%, with a mortality of 2 to 16%. The reported complications include a perforation rate of 4.2 to 10.5%, hemorrhage in 1.5 to 5%, tumor overgrowth in 8.5%, tube migration in 22%, and pressure necrosis of the esophageal wall in 4%.[29–34] The small luminal diameter leads to problems with food impaction in around 6.5%. The use of general anesthesia and the requirement for hospital admission also makes this treatment expensive.

Laser therapy has been shown in a number of studies to provide excellent palliation in malignant esophageal obstruction.[35–38] With the use of laser therapy, more than 80% of patients can be maintained on a solid or semisolid diet.[35–38] The main drawback of this modality is the requirement for multiple treatments, which must be repeated on a 4 to 8 times weekly basis. In a series of 189 patients with inoperable esophageal carcinoma, a mean of 3.3 procedures per patient was required.[37] The complication rate is low (5 to 9%)[35–38] and is mainly related to esophageal perforation due to pretreatment dilatation. The other main complication is hemorrhage, but this can be easily controlled by local laser photocoagulation.

Both laser therapy and self-expanding metal stents are used in our center for the palliation of malignant dysphagia. We have conducted a triple randomized study comparing Wall stents, Strecker stents, and laser therapy. The results demonstrated statistically significantly better palliation with metallic stents than with laser therapy.[39] However, there are certain morphologic types of tumor in which esophageal stents are best avoided. In situations where the tumor is very exophytic, or where the esophagus is very dilated above the stricture, the free end of the stent will not lie closely apposed to the esophageal wall, and food or fluid will tend to pool between the stent and the esophageal mucosa. In this situation, palliation will be suboptimal, and there is a risk of aspiration. We therefore find that esophageal stents and laser therapy are complementary treatments and that each case should be treated on its own merits.

Esophageal Stents in Benign Disease

In the majority of patients with malignant disease, the application of esophageal stents presents few long-term problems because most individuals have a fairly short survival. The management of benign disease is different, as in the long term one cannot be entirely certain about the difficulties that may be encountered. Generally we avoid the use of stents in this situation, but there are occasions when repeat dilatation produces progressively shorter periods of relief from dysphagia symptoms, in which there is little choice other than to employ a stent or submit the patient to major surgery. In addition, there are rare occasions when it is simply not possible to dilate benign strictures successfully. In general, we restrict the use of self-expanding stents in benign strictures to patients who are not fit for surgery. Clearly the use of a stent does not preclude surgery at a later date should that become necessary and should the patient's clinical condition improve sufficiently with adequate nutrition.

The technique for deploying esophageal stents across benign strictures is essentially the same as that in malignant disease, though we consider uncovered stents more appropriate as they are less likely to migrate, and in this clinical setting there is no potential for tumor ingrowth, making the stent covering superfluous. An additional advantage of using uncovered stents is that after a few months the stent is completely covered by epithelium and becomes incorporated into the wall of the esophagus. A number of cases involving the use of metallic stents in benign strictures are reported in the literature, and the results indicate a good response in terms of dysphagia.[40-44] However, the major problem in the long term is the occurrence of mucosal hypertrophy related to the stent (Fig. 2-5). This is usually amenable to balloon dilatation or laser treatment.

Treatment of Esophageal Leaks and Fistulae

Esophageal leaks or perforations may occur spontaneously (Boerhaave's syndrome) or following trauma, which may be iatrogenic (after balloon dilatation or surgery). Fistulae to the respiratory tract may be caused by a tumor arising either from the esophagus or from the tracheobronchial tree, or may be a complication of surgery or esophageal stenting.

Perforations and leaks are generally treated conservatively in the first instance, and most will heal if of benign origin. A proportion will be resistant, particularly if malignant in etiology, and in this situation the interventional radiologist can have an important role. The approach will depend on the underlying problem. In cases of malignancy, management is fairly straightforward, with deployment of a covered esophageal stent (Fig. 2-6). The published series describing treatment of malignant esophageal fistulae with covered self-expanding stents indicate a 95 to 100% success rate in covering the fistulae and preventing leakage into the mediastinum or the respiratory tract.[45-48]

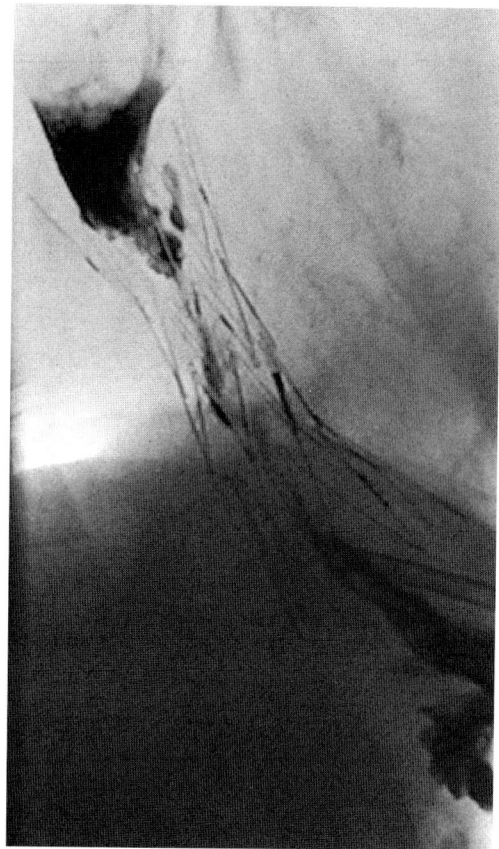

Figure 2-5 Patient had a modified Gianturco stent inserted for a resistant peptic stricture. This initially worked well, but subsequently recurrent dysphagia developed due to epithelial hyperplasia, as demonstrated on this esophagogram.

However, it should be noted that where a tracheoesophageal fistula lies very close to the crichopharyngeus, or where the esophagus is very dilated, use of a covered stent is likely to fail to seal the fistula. We have found the use of covered tracheal or bronchial stents useful in this situation (Fig. 2-7).

In patients with esophageal leaks from benign causes, such as Boerhaave's syndrome, the situation is less clear-cut. We have successfully used a covered Wallstent in this situation, though despite an initially impressive recovery, the patient died 8 weeks after stent insertion from a massive hematemesis.[49] We remain very conservative in the use of stents in this situation.

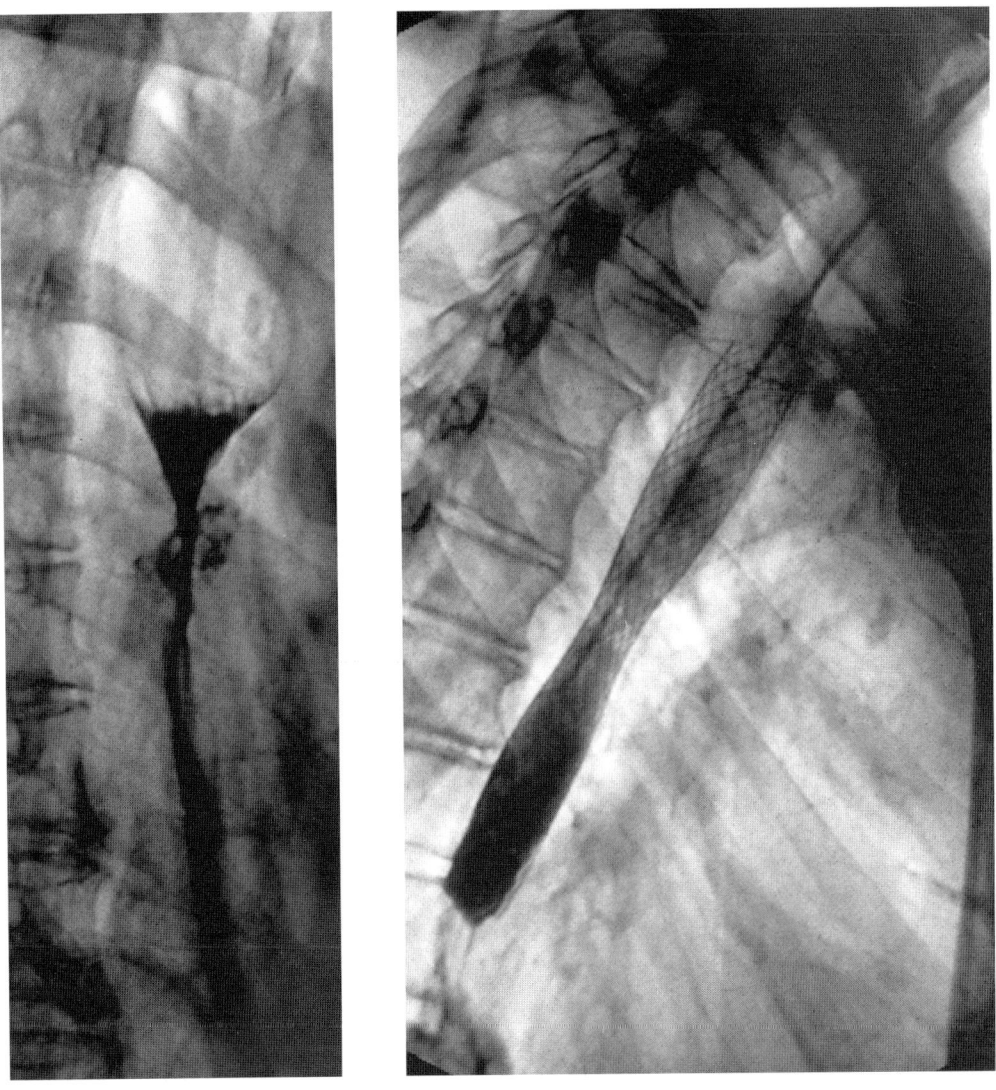

Figure 2–6 **(A)** A stricture with an associated leak due to squamous carcinoma. **(B)** After deployment of a covered Wallstent, the leak has healed. Note the residual waist on the stent.

Our preferred approach to the treatment of esophageal leaks of benign origin, after conservative treatment has failed, is the use of tissue adhesives, such as fibrin (Tisseel; Immuno, Toronto, Canada) or n-butyl-2-cyanoacrylate glue (Histoacryl; Davis and Geck, Gosport, Hants, UK). In the past this was performed endoscopically,[50,51] but more recently fluoroscopic guidance has been used.[52] The advantages of using fluoroscopic guidance rather than the endoscopic approach are avoidance of the risk of gluing the channel of the endoscope, and reduction in the degree of discomfort for the patient and the amount of sedation required. We have reported the use of n-butyl-2-cyanoacrylate glue for treatment of a fistula extending from a neoesophagojejunal anastomosis to the skin surface[53] and have more recently carried out with success two gluing procedures on postsurgical esophageal fistulae.

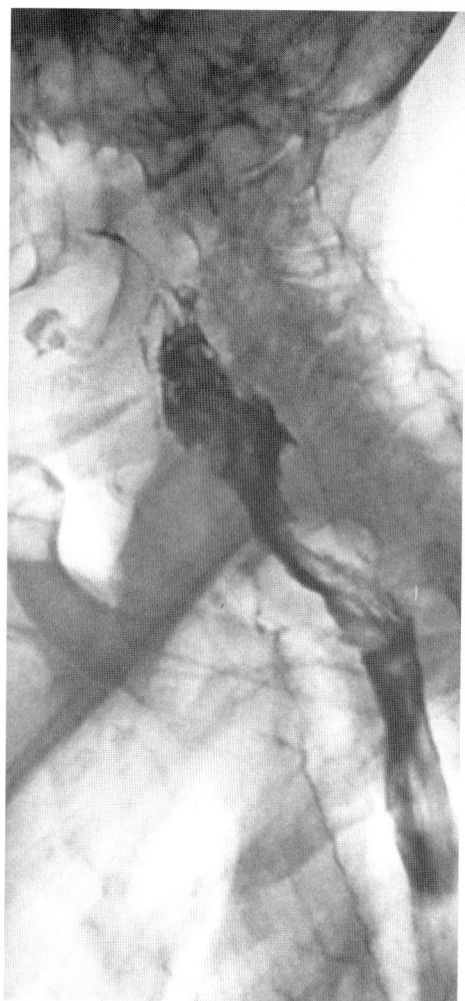 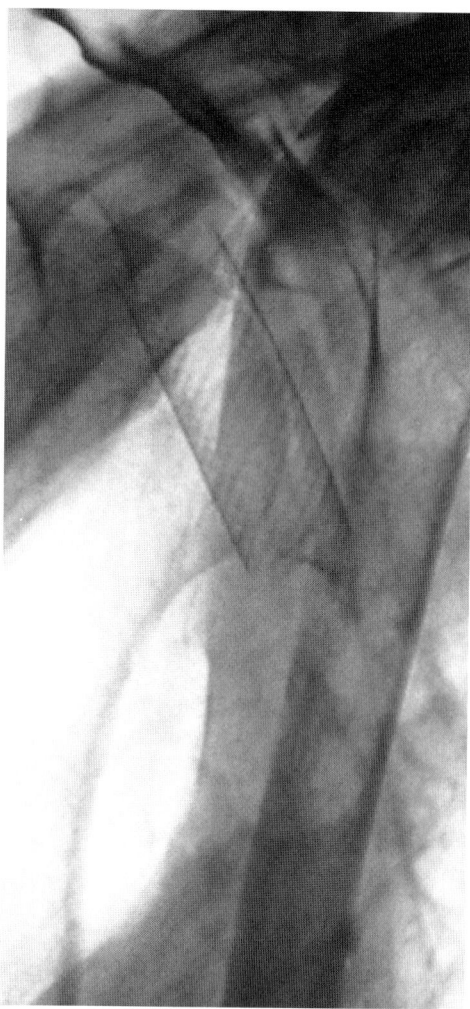

Figure 2–7 Patient had a tracheoesophageal fistula due to a squamous carcinoma. This caused minimal narrowing of the esophageal lumen. Upon endoscopic examinations the tumor was found to involve cricopharyngeus; therefore, an esophageal stent could not be employed. **(B)** An 18-mm-diameter covered tracheal stent was deployed to seal the fistula. After this there was no dysphagia and the symptoms of aspiration were relieved.

Radiologically guided closure of a duodenal fistula to the skin surface has also been described.[54] The variety of different fistulae tackled in this way also demonstrates the greater flexibility of the radiologic approach over endoscopy.

In the esophagus, the procedure begins with a contrast swallow to demonstrate the site and nature of the fistula. The patient then lies on the fluoroscopy table in the left lateral position, and the fistula is cannulated using a catheter and guide wire. The catheter tip is then placed in the proximal track. Two grams of monomeric *n*-butyl-2-cyanoacrylate is mixed with 2 mL of Lipiodol Ultrafluid (May & Baker Ltd, Dagenham, UK). The mixture is then injected rapidly from a plastic syringe and the catheter withdrawn immediately to prevent adhesion to the adjacent tissues.

We have encountered one patient who required several treatments, with the fistula improving after each one, indicating that if initial gluing fails, it may be worthwhile to persist. The application of glue is less likely to succeed in chronic fistulae that have become epithelialized. One group[54] describes tissue abrasion with a bronchial brush, which may help to overcome this. We have favored the use of n-butyl-2-cyanoacrylate, as it is more readily available, and there is no risk of infection, as may occur with concentrated blood products. However, fibrin does have the advantage that it is removed from the body by fibrinolysis over 4 to 6 weeks. Concerns have been raised about possible toxic side effects from n-butyl-2-cyanoacrylate.[53]

GASTRIC ANTRAL AND DUODENAL STENTING

Gastric outlet obstruction occurs most commonly secondary to malignancy arising either from the gastric antrum, or from duodenal stricture or obstruction secondary either to direct invasion or extrinsic compression or invasion from pancreatic carcinoma. Malignant strictures due to lymphoma or metastatic disease as well as benign lesions due either to chronic peptic ulceration or radiotherapy may also be encountered.

Many authors claim that the best palliative treatment for gastric outlet obstruction is a gastroenterostomy,[55] perhaps with the exception of lymphoma, where symptoms may be expected to improve with chemotherapy. However, even in these days of improved surgical results, a mortality rate of up to 14%[55] can be expected with palliative surgery. At present, stenting to relieve gastric outlet obstruction is generally only carried out in patients deemed unfit for surgery, but extension of their use is likely to occur in the next few years.

Insertion of stents via gastrostomy[56,57] or the peroral route has been described.[58-61] Endoscopy is frequently used but not strictly necessary,[61] although there is an absolute requirement for fluoroscopic screening. We favor the peroral route under fluoroscopic guidance. After the administration of intravenous sedation, a catheter and guide wire are passed through the esophagus down to the level of the stricture in either the gastric antrum or the duodenum. The catheter is manipulated across the stricture and the guide wire exchanged for an Amplatz superstiff exchange guide wire. The stricture is predilated to 10 mm in diameter, and an appropriate sized stent is deployed. A variety of stents have been used by different authors,[56-60] but we prefer the Wall stent because of its greater inherent outward radial force (Fig. 2-8). We use uncovered stents to minimize the risk of migration. We have used 16-mm-diameter stents,[61] which are probably the best compromise between a desirable large diameter and flexibility.

Results

Most published data are confined to case reports, all of which indicate technical success and good palliation of symptoms. The two series available, concerning 9[59] and 12[60] patients, respectively, indicate that immediate technical success can be expected in 89 to 100%, with successful palliation of symptoms in 78–100%. No major complications have been described, though one case of partial, asymptomatic stent migration was encountered by Binkert et al.[59] Given the relatively narrow stents that are used, soft diet is often advised, though frequently patients return to a normal diet of their own volition, and no evidence of food impaction has been encountered.[59] The reason for this is likely to be the somewhat more liquid nature of the gastric contents due to the action of gastric acid, making bolus impaction in stents at the gastric outlet less likely than if a similar sized stent were deployed in the esophagus. From the reports available in the literature, it is clear that patients recover very quickly after the procedure, and immediate palliation of their symptoms can be achieved. Therefore, we believe that there is now a case for more frequent use of stents as first-line palliation for malignant gastric outlet obstruction, as an alternative to

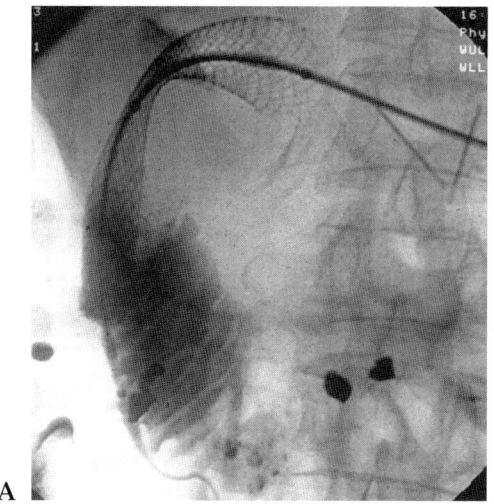 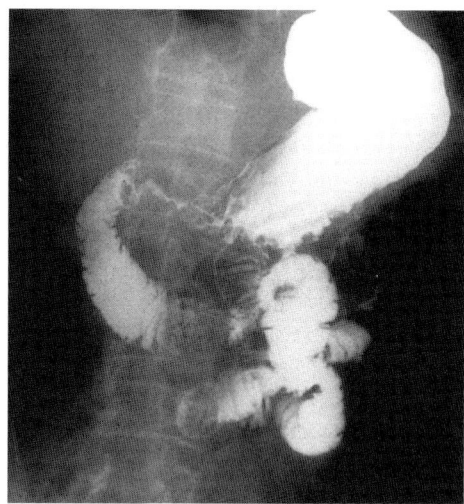

Figure 2–8 **(A)** Patient had developed gastric outlet obstruction due to an antral adenocarcinoma. **(B)** A 16-mm-diameter Wallstent was inserted and the patient's symptoms resolved. (Figure courtesy of Dr. A. J. Lopez.)

surgery, which continues to have a high mortality. This view is further reinforced by the fact that malignant biliary obstruction can be relieved almost without exception either percutaneously or endoscopically. It is now possible to palliate pancreatic carcinoma without recourse to surgery, with clear advantages for patients expected to survive for a relatively short period.

COLONIC STENTING

Colonic carcinoma is the most common tumor occurring in the United States, with 140,000 new cases diagnosed per year.[62] Conventional treatment is by surgical resection with or without chemotherapy, or if there is distant spread of disease some patients are treated with chemotherapy alone. Patients may present for the first time with acute large intestinal obstruction due to the tumor. Such patients are often in poor general condition and because of the obstruction cannot undergo preoperative bowel preparation. Therefore, treatment in this group usually involves an initial operation to fashion a defunctioning colostomy, with resection of the primary tumor. The distal bowel is left as a Hartman's pouch for later reanastomosis. Approximately 6 weeks later, an additional procedure to achieve reanastomosis of the bowel is undertaken. A two-stage approach is required because a primary anastomosis would fail in the presence of contaminated bowel. The major difficulty in performing emergency surgical treatment for acute malignant colonic obstruction is a reported mortality of up to 22%, compared with rates of 0.9 to 6.0% when surgery is carried out electively.[63,64] The ideal, therefore, is to avoid emergency surgery during acute obstruction. The use of rectosigmoid stenting facilitates this, allowing the patient's status to be optimized for an elective procedure, and allowing bowel preparation to take place prior to resection with a primary anastomosis.

Technique of Insertion

Having established that the patient has acute intestinal obstruction secondary to a malignant lesion, the patient is first rehydrated with an intravenous infusion, and a nasogastric tube is placed to decompress the bowel.

Access to the rectosigmoid region is gained with a sigmoidoscope, and a catheter and guide wire is passed through this and across the stricture. The stricture is then predilated to 15 mm, and an uncovered esophageal stent (20 to 22 mm diameter) is deployed across the strictured area. Esophageal stents have been used in the published series, but recently a dedicated rectosigmoid Wallstent has become available. An uncovered stent is employed to avoid problems with stent migration. Because in most cases the stent will be removed at surgical resection after bowel preparation, the potential for tumor ingrowth through the stent mesh is of little concern.

Results

Published reports indicate successful stent insertion in 91 to 100%,[65,66] with improvement in the obstructive picture within 48 hours in 83% and within 4 days in 100%.[66] Most patients undergo stenting followed by surgical resection of the primary tumor, but in patients unfit for surgery, stents are reported to provide good palliation.[66]

Potential complications include pain, migration, bleeding, and bowel perforation, though there are insufficient data to allow estimates of how common these may be.

Summary

Self-expanding metallic stents have been shown to be of great value in the palliation of malignant dysphagia and are superior to the other methods available, including laser therapy. The complications are minimal, but recurrent dysphagia due to tumor ingrowth and overgrowth continues to be a problem. This can be avoided by the use of covered stents in the upper two thirds of the esophagus, but to avoid problems with stent migration we no longer employ these stents at the gastroesophageal junction. It is at this site that ingrowth continues to be a problem, and new innovations will be required to combat this. Stents are used less frequently elsewhere in the GI tract but may be of use in the relief of gastric outlet obstruction and rectosigmoid colon tumors.

References

1. Earlam R. Esophageal cancer treatment in north east Thames region in 1981: medical audit using hospital activity analysis data. *Br Med J* 1984;288:1892–1894.
2. Parkin DM, Laara E, Muir CS. Estimates of the worldwide frequency of sixteen major cancers in 1980. *Int J Cancer* 1988;41:184–197.
3. Rankin S, Mason R. Staging of esophageal carcinoma. *Clin Radiol* 1992;46:373–377.
4. Cwiekiel W, Stridbeck H, Tranberg KG, et al. Malignant esophageal strictures: treatment with a self-expanding nitinol stent. *Radiology* 1993;187:661–665.
5. Saxon RR, Barton RE, Katon RM, et al. Treatment of malignant esophageal obstructions with covered metallic Z stents: long term results in 52 patients. *J Vasc Intervent Radiol* 1995;6:747–754.
6. Miyayama S, Matsui O, Kadoya M, et al. Malignant esophageal stricture and fistula: palliative treatment with polyurethane covered Gianturco stent. *J Vasc Intervent Radiol* 1995;6:243–248.
7. May A, Selmaier M, Hochberger J, et al. Memory metal stents for palliation of malignant obstruction of the esophagus and cardia. *Gut* 1995;37:309–313.
8. Song HY, Do YS, Han YM, et al. Covered, expandable esophageal metallic stent tubes: experiences in 119 patients. *Radiology* 1994;193:689–695.
9. Cowling MG, Hale H, Grundy A. The use of self-expanding metallic stents in the management of malignant oesophageal strictures. *Br J Surg* 1998;85:264–266.
10. Denton E, Morgan RA, Holemans J, et al. Metallic stents for the palliation of malignant dysphagia. *Br J Radiol* 1997;70(suppl):27.
11. Earlam R, Chunha-Melo JR. Esophageal squamous cell carcinoma: 1. A critical review of surgery. *Br J Surg* 1980;67:381–390.
12. Muller JM, Erasmi H, Stelzner M, et al. Surgical therapy of esophageal carcinoma. *Br J Surg* 1990;77:845–857.
13. Altorki NK, Girardi L, Skinner DB. Squamous cell carcinoma of the esophagus: therapeutic dilemma. *World J Surg* 1994;18:308–311.
14. Lerut TE, Leyn P, Coosemans W, et al. Advanced esophageal carcinoma. *World J Surg* 1994;18:379–387.
15. Earlam R, Chunha-Melo JR. Esophageal squamous cell carcinoma: 2. A critical review of radiotherapy. *Br J Surg* 1980;67:457–461.

16. Capsers RJL, Welvaart K, Verkes RJ, et al. The effect of radiotherapy on dysphagia and survival in patients with esophageal cancer. *Radiother Oncol* 1988;12:15–23.
17. Leslie MD, Dische S, Saunders MI, et al. The role of radiotherapy in carcinoma of the thoracic oesophagus: an audit of the Mount Vernon experience 1980–1989. *Clin Oncol* 1992; 4:114–118.
18. O'Rourke IC, Tiver K, Bull C, et al. Swallowing performance after radiation therapy for carcinoma of the esophagus. *Cancer* 1988;61:2022–2026.
19. Herskovic A, Martz K, Al-Sarraf M, et al. Combined chemotherapy and radiotherapy compared to radiotherapy alone in patients with cancer of the esophagus. *N Engl J Med* 1992;326:1593–1598.
20. Rowland CG, Pagliero KM. Intracavitary irradiation in palliation of carcinoma of the oesophagus and cardia. *Lancet* 1985;981–983.
21. Hishikawa Y, Kamikonya N, Tanaka S, et al. Radiotherapy of esophageal carcinoma: role of high dose rate intracavitary irradiation. *Radiother Oncol* 1987;9:13–20.
22. Harvey JC, Fleischman EH, Belloti JE, et al. Intracavitary radiation in the treatment of advanced esophageal carcinoma: a comparison of high dose rate vs. low dose rate brachytherapy. *J Surg Oncol* 1993;52:101–104.
23. Hishikawa Y, Tanaka S, Miura T. Esophageal ulceration induced by intracavitary irradiation for esophageal carcinoma. *Am J Roentgenol* 1984;143:269–273.
24. Herskovic A, Martz K, Al-Sarraf M, et al. Combined chemotherapy and radiotherapy compared to radiotherapy alone in patients with cancer of the oesophagus. *N Engl J Med* 1992;326:1593–1598.
25. Poplin EA, Khanuja PS, Kraut MJ, et al. Chemoradiotherapy of esophageal carcinoma. *Cancer* 1994;74:1217–1224.
26. Le Prise EA, Meunier BC, Etienne PL, et al. Sequential chemotherapy and radiotherapy for patients with squamous cell carcinoma of the esophagus. *Cancer* 1995;75:430–434.
27. Urba SG, Turrisi AT. Split-course accelerated radiation therapy combined with carboplatin and 5-fluorouracil for palliation of metastatic or unresectable carcinoma of the esophagus. *Cancer* 1995;74:435–439.
28. Coia LR, Soffen EM, Schultheiss TE, et al. Swallowing function in patients with esophageal cancer treated with concurrent radiation and chemotherapy. *Cancer* 1993;71: 281–286.
29. Tytgat GNJ. Endoscopic therapy of esophageal cancer: possibilities and limitations. *Endoscopy* 1990;22:263–267.
30. Den Hartog Jager FCA, Bartelsman JFWM, Tytgat GNJ. Palliative treatment of obstructing esophagogastric malignancy by endoscopic positioning of plastic a prosthesis. *Gastroenterology* 1979;77:1008–1014.
31. Gasparri G, Casalegno PA, Camadona M, et al. Endoscopic insertion of 248 prostheses in inoperable carcinoma of the esophagus and cardia: short-term and long-term results. *Gastrointest Endosc* 1987;33:354–356.
32. Fuegger R, Niederle B, Jantsch H, et al. Endoscopic tube implantation for the palliation of malignant esophageal stenosis. *Endoscopy* 1990;22:101–104.
33. Liakakos TK, Ohri SK, Townsend ER, et al. Palliative intubation for dysphagia in patients with carcinoma of the esophagus. *Ann Thorac Surg* 1992;53:460–463.
34. Spinelli P, Cerrai FG, Ciuffi M, et al. Endoscopic stent placement for cancer of the lower esophagus and gastric cardia. *Gastrointest Endosc* 1994;40:455–457.
35. Rau BK, Harikrishnan KM, Krishna S. Esophageal carcinoma: laser palliation in 231 cases. *Ann Acad Med Singapore* 1994;23: 32–34.
36. Sander RR, Poesl H. Cancer of the oesophagus—palliation—laser treatment and combined procedures. *Endoscopy* 1993;25 (suppl):679–682.
37. Mason RC, Bright N, McColl I. Palliation of malignant dysphagia with laser therapy: predictability of results. *Br J Surg* 1991;78: 1346–1347.
38. Maunoury V, Brunetaud JM, Cochelard D, et al. Endoscopic palliation for inoperable malignant dysphagia: long-term follow-up. *Gut* 1992;33:1602–1607.
39. Adam A, Ellul J, Watkinson AF, et al. Palliation of inoperable esophageal carcinoma: a prospective randomized trial of laser therapy and stent placement. *Radiology* 1997;202: 344–348.
40. Cwiekel W, Willen R, Stridbeck H, et al. Self expanding stent in the treatment of benign esophageal strictures: experimental study in pigs and presentation of clinical cases. *Radiology* 1993;187:667–671.

41. Foster DR. Use of a Strecker esophageal stent in the treatment of benign esophageal stricture. *Australasian Radiol* 1995;39:399–400.
42. Strecker E-R, Boos I, Vetter S, et al. Nitinol esophageal stents: new designs and clinical indications. *Cardiovasc Intervent Radiol* 1996;19:15–20.
43. Heindel W, Gossman A, Fischbach R, Michel O, Lackner K. Treatment of a ruptured anastomotic esophageal stricture following bougienage with a Dacron-covered nitinol stent. *Cardiovasc Intervent Radiol* 1996;19:431–434.
44. Tan B-S, Kennedy C, Morgan R, Owen W, Adam A. Uncovered metallic endoprostheses for recurrent benign esophageal strictures: preliminary experience. *Am J Roentgenol* 1997;169:1281–1284.
45. Morgan RA, Ellul JPM, Denton ERE, et al. Malignant esophageal fistulas and perforations: management with plastic-covered metallic endoprostheses. *Radiology* 1997;204:527–532.
46. Miyayama S, Matsui O, Kadoya M, et al. Malignant esophageal stricture and fistula: palliative treatment with polyurethane-covered Gianturco stent. *J Vasc Intervent Radiol* 1995;6:243–248.
47. Do YS, Song H-Y, Lee BH, et al. Esophagorespiratory fistula associated with esophageal cancer: treatment with a Gianturco stent tube. *Radiology* 1993;187:673–677.
48. Saxon RR, Barton RE, Katon RM, et al. Treatment of malignant esophagorespiratory fistulas with silicone covered metallic Z-stents. *J Vasc Intervent Radiol* 1995;6:237–242.
49. Adam A, Watkinson AF, Dussek J. Boerhaave syndrome: to treat or not to treat by means of insertion of a metallic stent. *J Vasc Intervent Radiol* 1995;6:741–746.
50. Kohler B, Kohler G, Reimann JF. Spontaneous esophagotracheal fistula resulting from ulcer in heterotopic gastric mucosa. *Gastroenterology* 1988;95:828–830.
51. Antonelli M, Cicconetti F, Vivino G, Gasparetto A. Closure of a tracheoesophageal fistula by bronchoscopic application of fibrin glue and decontamination of the oral cavity. *Chest* 1991;100:578–579.
52. Drury AE, Grundy A. Management of esophageal fistula by radiologically guided installation of tissue adhesive. *Clin Radiol* 1995;50:335–338.
53. Malcolm PN, Watkinson AF, Tan BS, Prasad P, Mason RC, Adam A. Radiological closure of an enteric fistula with *n*-butyl-2-cyanoacrylate—case report. *Minim Invasive Ther* 1996;5:571–574.
54. Brady AP, Malone DE, Tam P, McGrath FP. Closure of duodenal fistual with fibrin sealant. *J Vasc Intervent Radiol* 1993;4:525–529.
55. Watanapa P, Williamson RCN. Surgical palliation for pancreatic cancer: developments during the past two decades. *Br J Surg* 1992;79:8–20.
56. Keymling M, Wagner H-J, Vakil N, Knyrim K. Relief of malignant doudenal obstruction by percutaneous insertion of a metal stent. *Gastrointest Endosc* 1993;39:439–441.
57. Song H-Y, Yang D-H, Kuh J-H, Choi KC. Obstructing cancer of the gastric antrum: palliative treatment with covered metallic stents. *Radiology* 1993;187:357–358.
58. Solt J, Papp Z. Strecker stent implantation in malignant gastric outlet stenosis. *Gastrointest Endosc* 1993;39:442–443.
59. Binkert CA, Jost R, Steiner A, Zollikofer C. Benign and malignant stenoses of the stomach and duodenum: treatment with self-expanding metallic endoprostheses. *Radiology* 1996;199: 335–338.
60. Feretis C, Benakis P, Dimopoulos C, et al. Palliation of malignant gastric outlet obstruction with self-expanding metal stents. *Endoscopy* 1996;28:225–228.
61. Scott-Mackie P, Morgan R, Farrugia M, Glynos M, Adam A. Malignant duodenal obstruction: a role for metallic stents. *Br J Radiol* 1997;70:252–255.
62. Murray JJ. Colorectal cancer: principles of surgical resection. *Surg Clini North Am* 1993;73:103–116.
63. Witzig JA, Morel P, Erne M, Egeli R, Borst F, Rohner A. Chirgurie des cancers digestis les patients de plus de 80 ans. *Helv Chir Acta* 1993;59:767–769.
64. Messmer P, Thoni F, Ackermann C, Herzog U, Schuppissier J, Tondelli P. Perioperative morbidity and mortality of colon resection in colonic carcinoma. *Schweiz Med Wochenschr* 1992;122:1011–1014.
65. Rey J-F, Romanczyk T, Greff M. Metal stents for palliation of rectal carcinoma: a preliminary report on 12 patients. *Endoscopy* 1995;27:501–504.
66. Mainar A, Tejero E, Maynar M, Ferral H, Castaneda-Zuniga W. Colorectal obstruction: treatment with metallic stents. *Radiology* 1996;198:761–764.

Chapter 3

Percutaneous Gastrostomy, Gastroenterostomy, and Jejunostomy

David D. Kidney
Larry-Stuart Deutsch

In 1822, Alexis St. Martin, a French–Canadian fur trapper, was injured by a musket in the left flank. At the time, Dr. William Beaumont, a U.S. Army surgeon, wrote:

> *I found a portion of the lung, as large as a turkey's egg, protruding through the external wound, lacerated and burnt; and immediately below this, another protrusion which, on examination, proved to be a portion of the stomach, lacerated through all its coats, and pouring out the food he had taken for his breakfast through an orifice large enough to admit the forefinger.*[1,2]

Based on this fortuitous accident and the resultant natural window, or traumatic percutaneous gastrostomy, Beaumont performed numerous experiments. Many of his conclusions about gastric physiology and secretion have stood the test of time and been confirmed by modern methods. Gastrostomy has since gained popularity and is now a widely accepted method for providing nutritional support or bowel decompression in a wide range of clinical scenarios.

The idea of gastrostomy as a means of delivering nutritional support was conceived by Egeberg, a Norwegian surgeon, in 1841.[3] The first successful gastrostomy was performed by Verneuil in Paris in 1876.[4] Surgical gastrostomy remained the only option until 1979, when Gauderer and Ponsky performed a forced percutaneous endoscopic gastrostomy (PEG).[5,6] Radiologic fluoroscopic-guided percutaneous gastrostomy is the newest gastrostomy technique; it was originally performed by Preshaw in 1981.[7] All three methods continue to be widely used, though the nonsurgical methods are gaining acceptance due to decreased morbidity and cost.

Modifications to the surgical placement and operative gastrostomy were introduced in 1839 by Sedillot. The operative and surgical technique has been modified and tailored over the years by Woodsoe (1891), Stamm (1894), and Dupage and Janeway (1913).[8] Recently, laparoscopy has been used during surgical gastrostomy.[9,10]

PEG placements also have been modified. The original Ponsky "pull" technique, the Sachs-Vine "push-through" technique, and the Russell "push introducer" method[5,6,11,12] all continue to find use, each with its own proponents.

INDICATIONS

The provision of enteral nutritional support remains the most common indication for gastrostomy, as gastrostomies are rarely placed for bowel decompression. The use of enteral nutrition in hospitals is increasing, especially in critically ill patients. Typical patients are those with neurologic disease secondary to cerebrovascular accidents, trauma, or neurosurgery, and those with obstructive dysphagia secondary to tumor. Increased use has led to an expanding role for physicians, gastroenterologists, surgeons, and radiologists who can provide enteral access.

A large number of patients whose gastrointestinal tract functions normally may not be capable of eating because of various physiologic or anatomical difficulties with the swallowing mechanism. In these cases, short-term nutritional support has been delivered through the presence of nasogastric (NG) feeding tubes, which are now soft, small-bore catheters. They have problems of increased gastroesophageal reflux with the potential for aspiration, pharyngeal irritation, and peptic esophagitis, which are major causes of patient dissatisfaction. In two recent studies comparing percutaneous gastrostomy and NG feeding in a group of stroke patients, outcomes measured by clinical improvement mortality and nutritional state were superior with percutaneous gastrostomy and were more acceptable to patients.[13,14]

Early feeding in critically ill patients has become more prevalent and popular.[15] Malnutrition is significant in U.S. hospital patients.[16] In a critically ill patient, such as a postsurgical patient, it is now accepted that an early feeding jejunostomy can permit immediate postoperative enteral feeding even in the absence of detectable bowel sounds.[17] The advantages of enteral over parenteral feeding in the nutritionally depleted patient is well established. Enteral feeding is safer, easier to administer, has more physiologic beneficial effects on the bowel, and is less expensive.[18,19] A further advantage of enteral over parenteral nutritional support is the beneficial effect on the intestinal histology and structure in addition to the immunonutritional status of the patient. Enteral nutrition has the potential to decrease infective wound complications, reducing the need for antibiotic coverage and shortening hospitalization.[20]

Patients with Crohn's disease, small bowel syndromes, or impaired small bowel absorption benefit from enterally administered elemental diets. The complicated cardiac surgery patient, the patient with pancreatitis, the patient with cirrhosis who is malnourished, and other patients who need organ-specific enteral support also benefit.[21,22]

The use of gastrostomy or gastrojejunostomy (GJ) for decompression is a well-recognized practice, but the frequency of usage depends largely on the patient population. These techniques are most commonly performed in patients with carcinomatosis for the purpose of bowel decompression, thus eliminating the need for long-term nasogastric suction. Initially, a number of authors recommend the use of large-bore (24- to 28-Fr) catheters, though smaller catheters have been shown to achieve similar results.[23–25]

Once one has decided on a percutaneous approach, the next decision lies between a gastric or jejunal location of the feeding tube tip, that is, a gastrostomy or a GJ placement.[25] The controversy between jejunal and gastric tip placement is largely based on the risk of reflux and aspiration. Clearly, patients who are refluxing and aspirating benefit from transpyloric jejunal tube placement. Placement of the catheter tip beyond the ligament of Treitz reduces the risk of gastroesophageal reflux to virtually zero.[26,27] However, placement of a jejunal tube does have one drawback: physiologically, a jejunostomy feeding tube requires a longer and slower infusion time, whereas with the gastrostomy tube (G tube) simple bolus feeding is feasible.

There are two approaches to this particular problem: One may choose to place GJ tubes in all patients,[25] or one can select specific patients who are at increased risk, such as those with a documented history of reflux aspiration, with elevated gastric residual, or for whom reflux aspiration would be catastrophic.[28,29] Most physicians use common sense and clinical judgment on a patient-to-patient basis in deciding whether to place a G or a GJ tube.

CONTRAINDICATIONS

As more experience is gained and as radiologists become more comfortable with percutaneous techniques, the number of relative and absolute contraindications to percutaneous gastrostomy diminishes.

Some "absolute" contraindications, when reviewed on an individual basis, may in reality be a feasible and safe option. These include patients with total gastrectomy, carcinoma involving all of the gastric wall, or extensive gastric varices. In the presence of a total gastrectomy it may be feasible to place a percutaneous jejunostomy tube (Figs. 3–1 and 3–2).[30–32] In patients with gastric carcinomatosis, problems include picking a safe site (due to the risk of hemorrhage) and accomplishing gastric distention. If gastric varices are extensive, identification of a safe puncture site is the critical deciding factor. If an appropriate site can be identified, possibly with computed tomography (CT) or ultrasonography, percutaneous or endoscopic methods remain appropriate.[24]

Relative contraindications include bleeding diathesis and an unsatisfactory access route to the stomach secondary to massive hepatomegaly, or interposed colon or ascites. Interposition of colon is a significant problem, but some manipulation with complete distention of the stomach or placement of a rectal tube may move the transverse colon out of the access plane. An infracolic route may also be used.[33] When the liver is enlarged, it is not ideal to traverse that organ for the placement of a gastrostomy tube but it is possible to traverse a small portion of liver without adverse sequellae.[32] Coagulopathies must be reversed prior to percutaneous gastrostomy, whereas ascites can be dealt with using a combination of preprocedure drainage and gastropexy.

Technique and Materials

Currently, three distinct methods of gastrostomy are available: surgical, endoscopic (PEG), and percutaneous (PG). The trend has been toward nonsurgical gastrostomy because the surgical methods are carried out predominantly under general anesthesia and have a significant associated morbidity.[34] Percutaneous gastrostomy with fluoroscopic guidance has been shown to be safe and effective.[24,25,35–43]

Preprocedure

Once the appropriateness of the procedure as the method of choice for nutritional support or bowel decompression has been established, a directed medical history, physical examination, and review of pertinent imaging must be completed. Important information, such as history of previous abdominal surgery or presence of organomegaly, may become apparent during this review. Any evidence of a bleeding abnormality should trigger an investigation and any revealed coagulopathy should be corrected prior to the procedure.

The patient must fast overnight and an NG tube should be placed, if possible. If there is difficulty in placing the NG tube due to patient intolerance or the presence of an obstructive lesion, this step can be deferred until the patient is in the interventional suite. We depend on a review of previous imaging studies and fluoroscopic assessment of the upper abdomen to check for interposition of colon or liver between the desired entry site and stomach. Some authors recommend sonographic evaluation of the liver and liver edge marking on the patient's abdomen. Some authors also administer oral barium on the evening before the study or a limited enema at the time of the procedure for the purpose of outlining the colon.[24,25,40] In our institution, with a directed physical examination, review of imaging studies, and fluoroscopic assessment of the location of both colon and liver edge, we feel confident when excluding significant organomegaly or organ displacement along the proposed puncture path.[29]

Procedure

All of our procedures are performed under fluoroscopic guidance with the patient supine and the left upper quadrant prepped and draped in a sterile fashion. We achieve adequate anesthesia with local anesthetic, which we supplement with intravenous morphine and midazolam to achieve conscious sedations with pertinent physiologic monitoring.

If an NG tube is present, we proceed to inflate the stomach and then select an ideal skin puncture site. If the patient has an obstructive lesion or other difficulty affecting

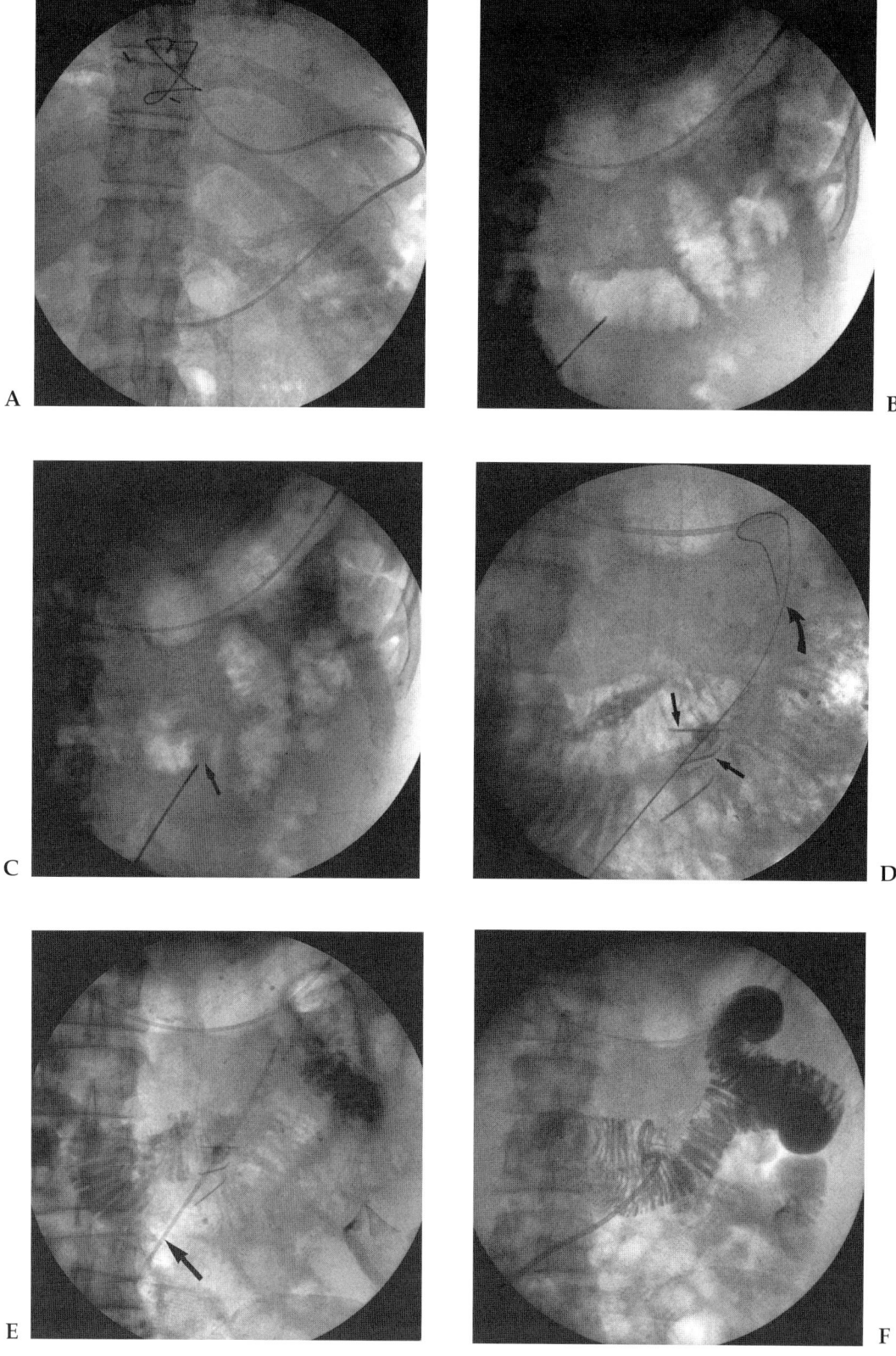

NG tube placement, then we attempt to traverse the obstruction using guide wire and catheter techniques under fluoroscopic guidance. We typically use a multipurpose catheter (Cook, Inc., Bloomington, IN) and a Bentson guide wire (Cook, Inc.). When this maneuver is unsuccessful, we inflate the stomach directly via a 22-gauge Chiba needle placed percutaneously directly into the stomach bubble. Once access has been obtained, the stomach is distended with air and a puncture site chosen (Fig. 3–3B). Some authors advocate administering 0.5 mg of intravenous glucagon for bowel paresis in all cases, but we tend to use it only when we are having difficulty in maintaining adequate gastric distention.[24,43]

Most radiologists use a modification of the Seldinger technique for the placement of their G tube; however, a one-step trocar method involving a single puncture has also been described.[5,6] We puncture in a left subcostal position at or just lateral to the lateral margin of the rectus muscle to avoid the inferior epigastric artery and vein, following administration of sufficient local anesthetic and 1-cm skin incision. We use an 18-gauge needle and advance a 0.38-inch Coons guide wire (Cook, Inc.) (Fig. 3–3C,D). Smaller needles have been used, but we like the stiffness of the 18-gauge for puncturing the thick gastric wall. With respect to the ideal puncture site, most people choose a mid- or distal gastric body site, preferably equidistant between the lesser and greater curvatures. This choice of puncture site is an attempt to avoid the major arterial branches supplying the stomach from the left and right gastroepiploic artery and the left gastric artery. We puncture angling medially so that the track will facilitate easy access to the pylorus for potential GJ tube placement. It is critical that this puncture be observed with fluoroscopy because one must be certain that the first viscus indented by the needle is indeed the stomach, not the colon or small bowel, and then a jabbing motion, rather than a gradual pushing motion, is used to puncture the thick muscular gastric wall.

Once access to the stomach lumen has been gained and the guide wire placed, the tract is typically sequentially dilated and the gastrostomy catheter placed over the guide wire. In our institution, our technique has evolved from our previous published data[29] when we used sequential dilatation, using a peel-away sheath with a 16-Fr catheter placed over the guide wire via the peel-away sheath. We presently use the Deutsch gastrostomy catheter, a modified 16-Fr Cope-loop G tube with hydrophilic coating and extralarge sideholes (Cook, Inc.). This is advanced directly over the guide wire, with the metal stiffener in place until the gastric lumen has been reached. The catheter is then further advanced over the guide wire with a jabbing motion while the stiffener is held rigid (Fig. 3–3F). With the appropriate hydrophilic coating and gastric distention to ensure an appropriate counterforce, this technique is now quicker, easier, and more successful, and it reduces the number of steps and potential errors. At the conclusion of the procedure we confirm the intragastric position by an injection of

Figure 3–1 A 52-year-old man with end-stage pulmonary disease and ischemic cardiomyopathy in need of nutritional support. Jejunostomy was chosen due to high risk of aspiration. **(A)** Multipurpose catheter advanced with tip in the proximal duodenum. **(B)** Following air insufflation, an appropriate jejunal loop is identified. **(C)** Initial percutaneous puncture. The bowel wall is displaced by the puncture needle (*arrow*). **(D)** Following the deployment of fasteners (*arrows*), a guide wire is advanced (*curved arrow*). **(E)** The tract is sequentially dilated (*arrow*). **(F)** A 12-Fr Cope loop catheter is advanced, reformed, and the position confirmed by contrast medium injection.

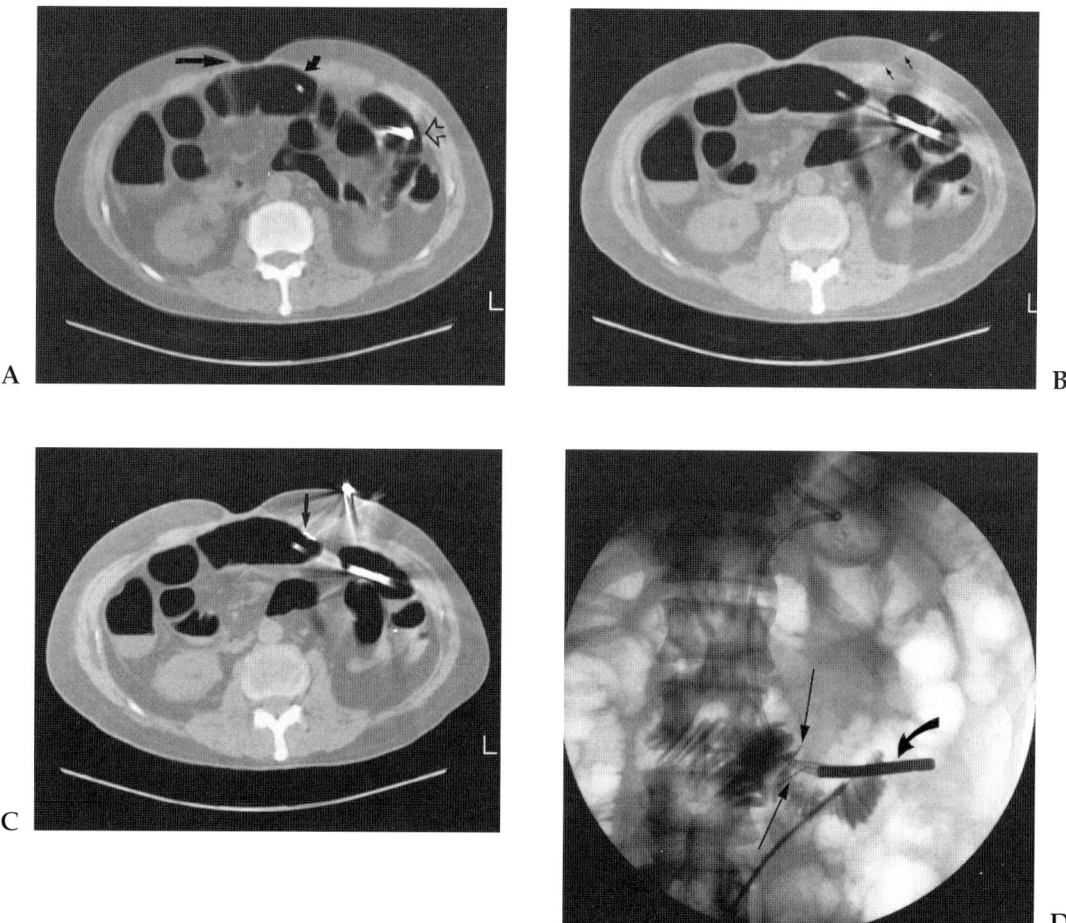

Figure 3–2 A 50-year-old man following gastrectomy for carcinoma. Jejunostomy was requested for nutritional support. **(A)** CT scan shows surgical defect (*arrow*) and distended small bowel loop immediately adjacent to anterior abdominal wall (*curved arrows*). Tip of nasojejunal tube is also seen (*open arrow*). **(B)** CT scan shows needle (*small arrows*) tract through significant soft tissue to the bowel lumen. **(C)** CT scan shows a T fastener (*arrow*) in place opposing the anterior bowel wall to the anterior abdominal wall. **(D)** Fluoroscopic image shows two gastropexy devices (arrows), nasojejunal-tube (*curved arrow*), 0.18 guide wire and dilator in situ with contrast injection to confirm intraluminal location. **(E)** The tract is sequentially dilated and a Coons guide wire advanced (*arrow*). **(F)** A 16-Fr hydrophilic G tube is advanced with the stiffener in place (*arrow*). **(G)** The G tube is advanced alone over the guide wire. **(H)** The catheter loop is formed and contrast medium injected to confirm location.

contrast (Fig. 3–3H). We do not suture or place any kind of retention device at the skin surface, preferring to allow a certain amount of freedom for movement at the skin entrance.

Postprocedure

We allow the gastrostomy to be used once normal bowel sounds are noted. The feedings are titrated to full strength by the

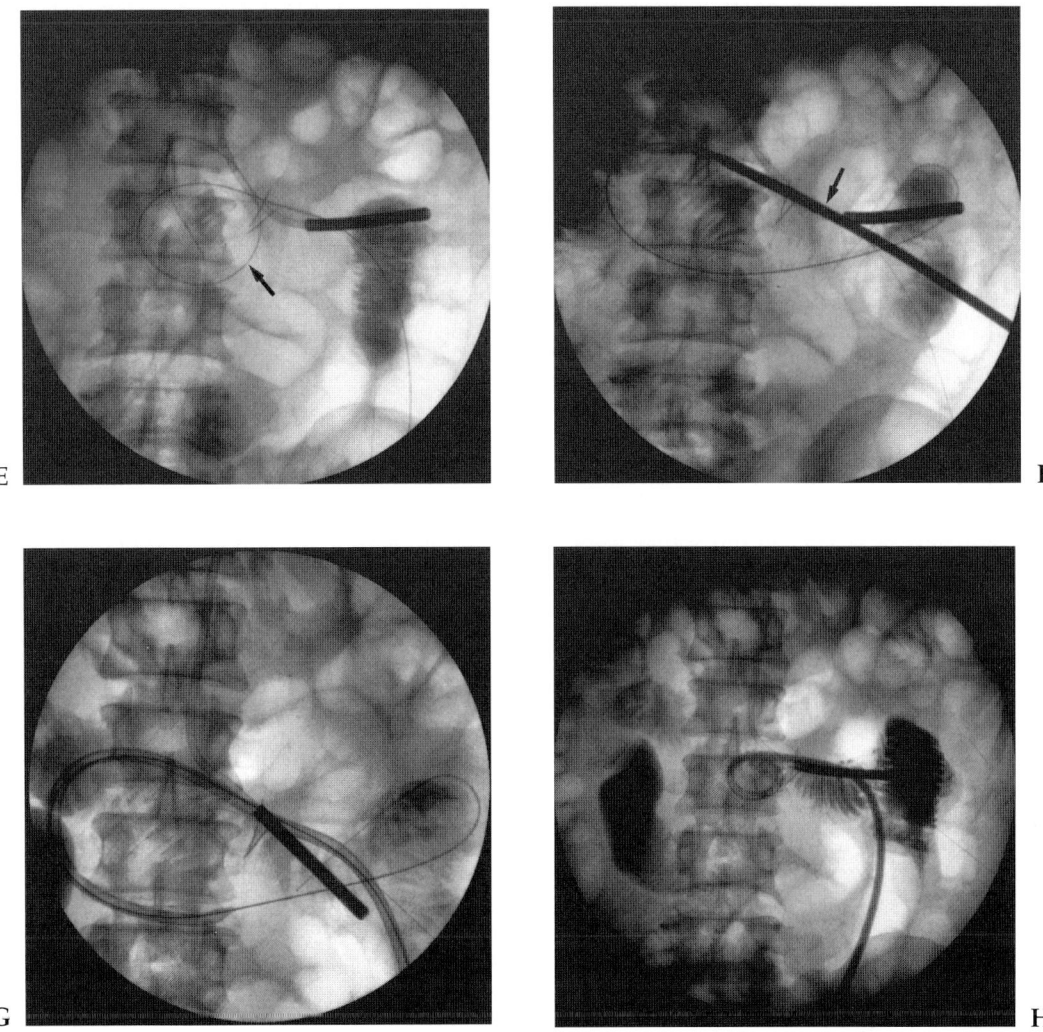

Figure 3–2 *(Continued)*

dietician. We allow only liquids to be given via the G tubes and advocate the use of liquid medication formulations. The G tubes are replaced as an outpatient procedure in the interventional radiology suite at 6-month intervals, or earlier if they become clogged or displaced.

In patients who are confused or at risk for accidental removal of their tube, we employ some type of abdominal binder to discourage catheter removal, particularly during the first week, in addition to the possible deployment of gastropexy devices.

Whether some from of gastropexy is necessary in percutaneous gastrostomy remains controversial.[24,29,39,44] The devices used are the Cook Cope suture anchor (Cook, Inc., Bloomington, IN) and the MediTech nylon T fastener (MediTech Corp., Watertown, MA). The devices are similar, consisting of a short metal bar with a suture attached at midpoint. They are mounted in an 18-gauge needle and deployed in the gastric lumen after the gastric wall has been punctured with a pushing wire. With gentle traction on the suture the short bar anchors the gastric wall

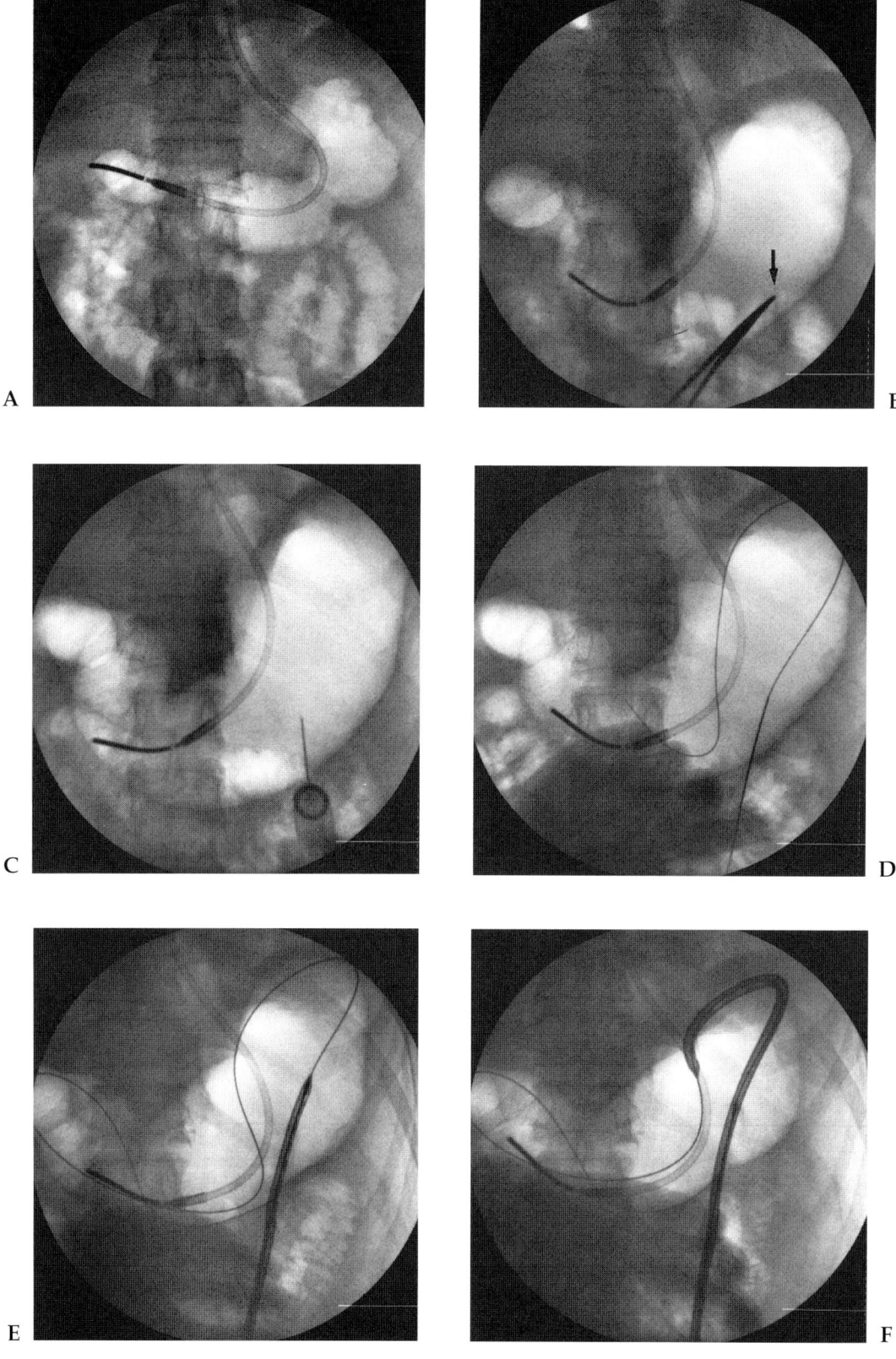

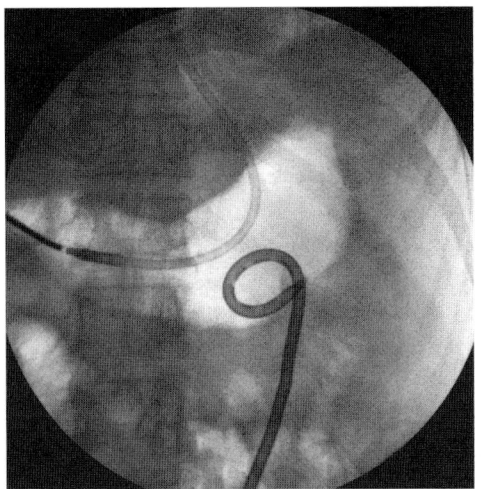
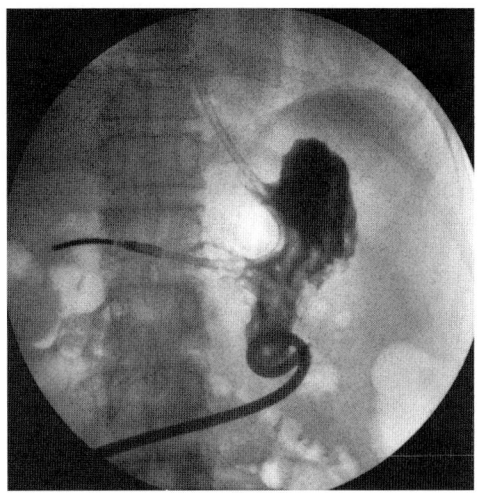

Figure 3–3 A 78-year-old man, following cerebrovascular accident, in need of gastrostomy tube placement for nutritional support. A series of eight images demonstrating G-tube placement. **(A)** tube is in place without evidence of interposed liver or colon. **(B)** Stomach is inflated and appropriate site for puncture noted (*arrow*). **(C)** Initial puncture with 18-gauge puncture needle is followed by **(D)** rapid advancement of guide wire into gastric lumen. **(E)** A 16-Fr catheter and stiffener combination is advanced to the gastric lumen. **(F)** Catheter is advanced with the stiffener held rigid. **(G)** Stiffener and guide wire are removed and the catheter is reformed. **(H)** Contrast injection confirms intraluminal gastric location.

to the abdominal wall; then the sutures are secured to the skin. As many as four gastropexy devices are used by some operators. The suture is typically cut once a tract has formed at 2 to 3 weeks. The point of gastropexy is to prevent leakage into the peritoneal cavity and to ensure the formation of a fibrous tract to decrease complications.[39] We believe that the routine use of gastropexy fixation before percutaneous gastrostomy in the adult patient is not warranted because of the lack of clinical proven benefit. The stomach wall is composed of three thick muscular layers that are oriented at oblique angles to one another and form an extremely tight seal around the gastrostomy catheter, which we feel is adequate to prevent significant leakage. Saini et al propose further possible benefit of gastropexy; they believe that an element of tamponade may be achieved to prevent significant hemorrhage from a possible arterial injury.[39] However, the addition of further needle punctures should increase the risk of hemorrhage to a greater degree than the proposed reduction by the placement of these T fasteners.

We do use gastropexy devices, T fasteners, or T tacks in specific situations. We typically place fasteners in patients who are at increased risk for accidental removal or who may be confused or combative, in patients with a significant volume of ascites to prevent leakage of acidic fluid around the puncture site, and for direct percutaneous jejunostomy or gastrostomy in patients following gastric surgery.[45]

Spillage of gastric juices into the abdominal cavity is most likely to occur during dilatation of the tract to the stomach. Therefore, it is imperative that the operator identify the invagination or visible puckering of the stomach wall as the various dilator or peel-away sheath systems are advanced. One common problem is with intraperitoneal or intramural coiling of guide wires of catheters. The gastric wall is sufficiently resistant to penetration that invagination of the visceral wall during tract dilatation can be mistaken for traversal which, to the inexperienced eye, may appear to be intragastric and result in extraluminal deployment of the catheter. This point cannot be overemphasized, particularly when one is teaching or demonstrating the technique to residents and fellows.

Gastrojejunostomy Tubes

Documented aspiration is a clear indication for advancement of the tip of the feeding catheter to the jejunum. Aspiration is an extremely serious complication, with a mortality of 43% noted in Light's series among patients who had aspiration after PEG.[46] There are a number of potential disadvantages of GJ tubes that must be considered prior to their placement. Technically, the procedure is more difficult and has a slightly higher technical failure rate than simple gastrostomy (2.8% in Bell's series).[25] The feeding regimen is different, necessitating longer and slower feedings to prevent diarrhea; however, overall a satisfactory regimen may consist of just four 60-minute feedings each day. These GJ tubes also are longer and tend to have smaller lumens and therefore an increased risk of clogging.[47]

In the placement of percutaneous gastrojejunostomy (PGJ) tubes the technique is similar to that of percutaneous gastrostomy (Fig. 3–4). It is a personal preference whether one places gastropexy devices, but there are advantages to the placement of PGJ tubes. In addition to opposing the gastric wall to the abdominal wall, they provide countertraction during manipulation of catheters and dilatation of the tract to prevent invagination of the gastric wall and buckling of the device in the peritoneal cavity. Once access to the gastric lumen has been gained, the pylorus is negotiated with a suitable catheter and guide wire and advanced to the jejunum beyond the ligament of Treitz. If this is being done de novo, the critical point is to ensure that the initial gastric puncture tract is angled toward the pylorus. Once this is achieved, a guide wire and catheter combination can be manipulated to traverse the pylorus and advanced to the jejunum with relative ease. It is then possible to place the GJ tube over the stiff guide wire that is in place.

When converting a G tube to a GJ tube, the tract is usually cranial or lateral in orientation, which makes the negotiation of catheter and guide wire to the pylorus much more difficult.[48,49] This is particularly common when the G tube was initially placed by an alternate method, either surgical or endoscopic. In either case, we have found that when there is a difficulty with the catheter and guide wire coiling in the gastric fundus, advancing a stiff sheath or dilator and manipulating the tract provides the best chance of directing the system toward the pylorus.[50] As a last resort, one can leave the G tube in place and use a new puncture for the GJ tube. This may be a realistic option in patients in whom a short procedure time is critical and lengthy procedures and manipulations are potentially risky.

One should note the size and type of catheter and, if it is to be removed, ensure that the new GJ catheter is of a similar or larger size to prevent peritubal leakage. In surgically placed catheters, we have on occasion been able to advance a single-lumen jejunal feeding tube through the surgical gastrostomy, thus reducing both procedure time and difficulty.[51]

When dealing with a PEG, the first problem is to deal with the rigid bumper at the end of PEG tubes. One can simply cut the catheter close to the skin and allow the bumper to pass through the gastrointestinal tract, a method that, as described by Burdick et al, can cause symptoms of small bowel obstruction.[52] Alternatively, one can

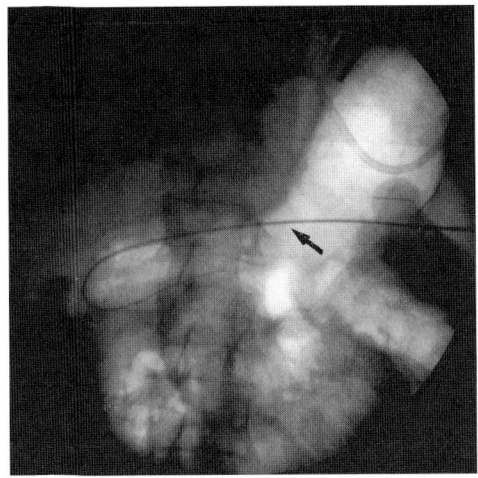
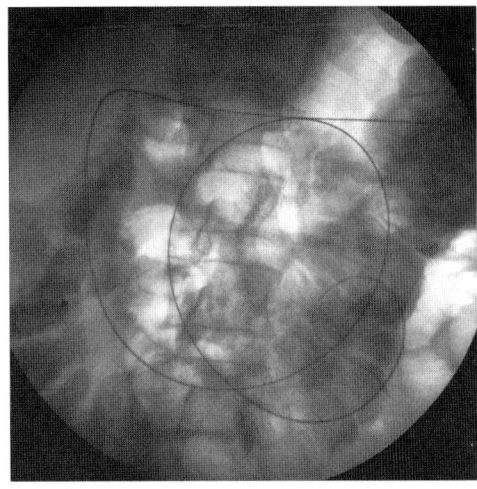
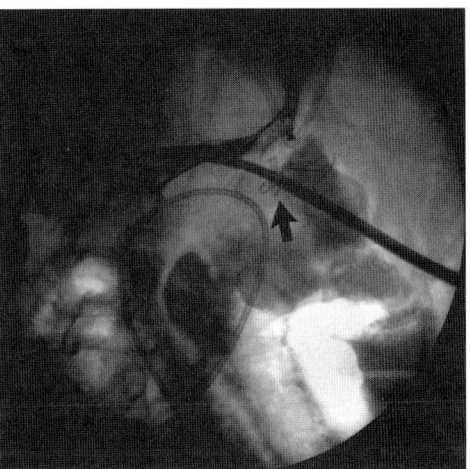

Figure 3–4 A 38-year-old man who is HIV-positive, with significant respiratory compromise and at high risk for aspiration, in need of gastrojejunostomy for nutritional support. **(A)** With puncture toward the pylorus, catheter and guide wire are advanced (*arrow*). **(B)** Guide wire and catheter are advanced to the jejunum. **(C)** Malecot device forms in gastric lumen (*arrow*).

attempt to retrieve the bumper endoscopically, which defeats the purpose of trying to do the procedure radiologically or with fluoroscopic guidance. We have occasionally cut the catheter close to the skin and advanced an angiographic guide wire up the esophagus to the mouth and externally. With control of both ends of the wire, the bumper stump is tied with a loop suture to the abdominal end of the guide wire, thus allowing the wire with bumper attached to be removed via the oral cavity (Fig. 3–5). At all times a second safety guide wire is in place in the stomach to maintain tract access. A second but more expensive method that we have used is to advance a nitinol snare and guide wire to the stomach from the mouth and retrieve the bumper stump in that fashion.

Materials

There is an overwhelming array of G tubes and a more manageable number of GJ catheters available on the market. Initially, a simple Foley catheter was the most commonly used catheter, but problems with deflation and accidental removal have brought about their replacement by more specific catheters with a variety of fixation techniques. Modifications have advanced significantly since the initial use of Foley-type balloon catheters. Several self-locking or friction lock–type catheters that have

CHAPTER 3 · Percutaneous Gastrostomy, Gastroenterostomy, and Jejunostomy

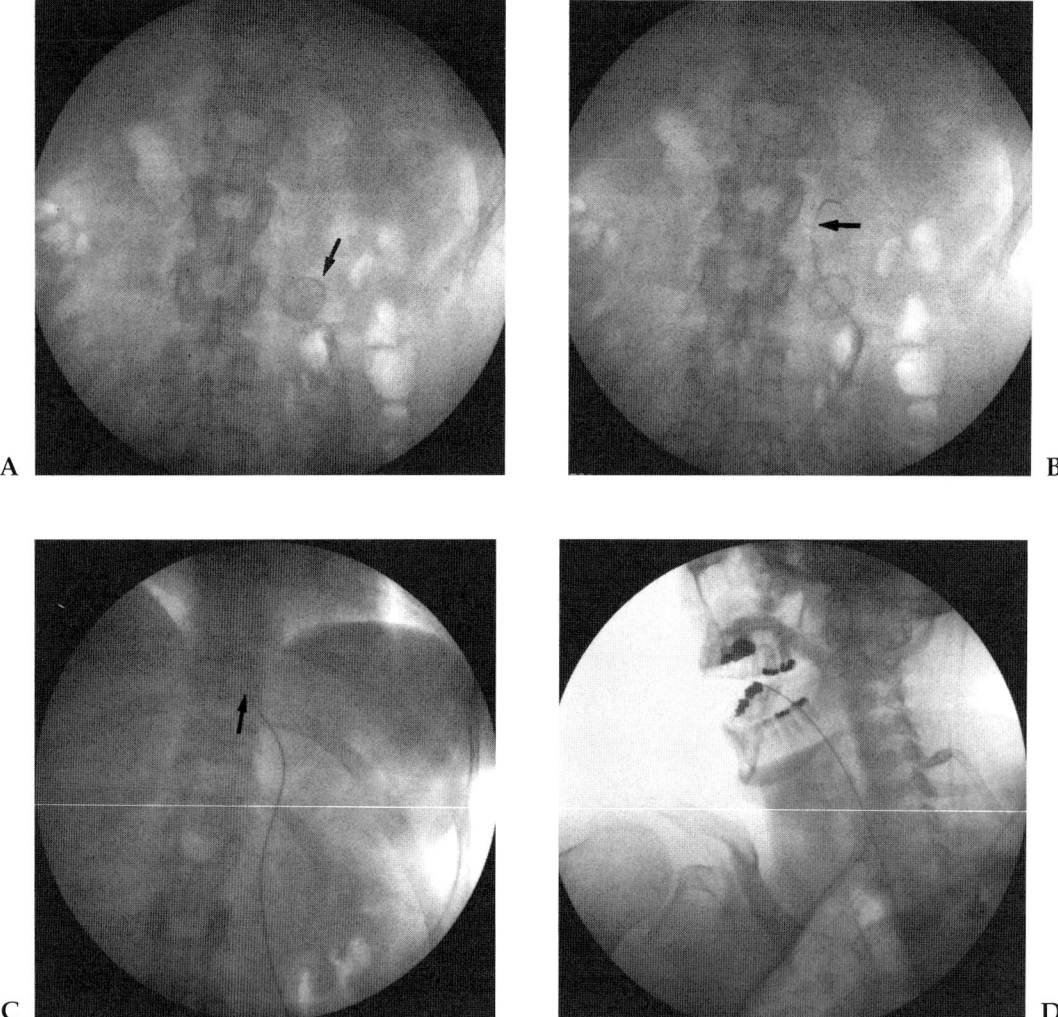

Figure 3–5 A 36-year-old woman. **(A)** Initial image shows percutaneous endoscopic gastrostomy (PEG) catheter in place (*arrow*). **(B)** Advancement of catheter through the PEG (*arrow*). **(C)** Reverse esophageal catheterization with the guide wire (*arrow*). **(D)** Advancement of guide wire to the mouth for subsequent peroral PEG removal.

been used by interventional radiologists in other countries are now being used in the United States. It is largely a matter of personal preference which catheter is placed, but several parameters should be considered. First, the lumen must be large enough for feeding and decompression when required yet small enough to prevent unnecessary patient discomfort. Second, various catheter terminations are available to aid in gastric retention, each with its own stated advantages (e.g., Cope loop, Malecot, and balloon devices).

All the major companies have a number of G tubes and GJ tubes that cover all possible variables and eventualities. We use the Deutsch gastrostomy catheter (a 16-Fr self-retaining Cope loop hydrophilic

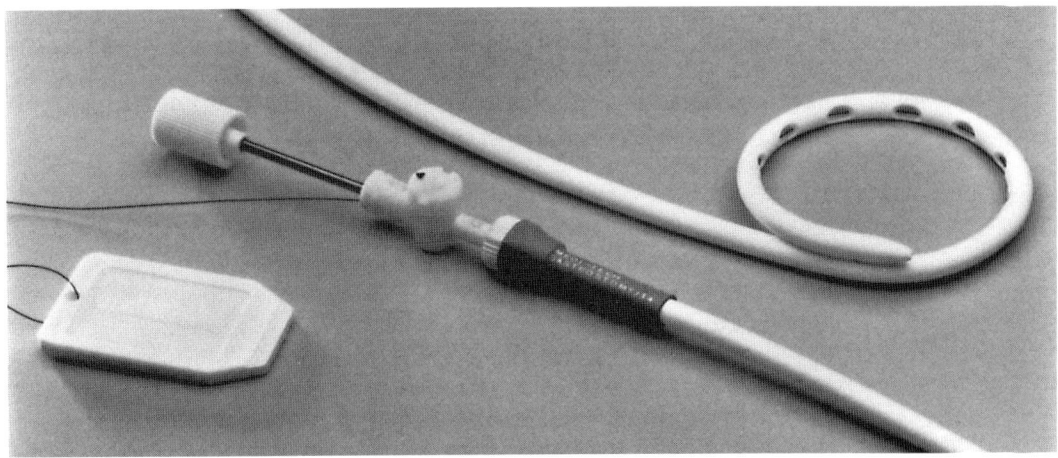

Figure 3–6 The vanSonnenberg gastrostomy catheter (MediTech, Watertown, MA), 14 Fr with a self-locking loop.

gastrostomy catheter; Cook, Inc.), but also available are the Wilms-Oglesby gastrostomy (Cook, Inc.) and the vanSonnenberg gastrostomy catheters (MediTech), which are 14 Fr with self-locking loops (Fig. 3–6). The Deutsch catheter is a modified polyurethane catheter whose hydrophilic coating decreases its coefficient of friction by 86%, thus permitting single-step placement without the need for either gastropexy or tract dilatation (Fig. 3–7).

When considering a GJ tube, one also must consider a single lumen catheter, such as the Shetty tube (Cook, Inc.), or a double-lumen catheter, which gives one the option of simultaneous gastric aspiration. A double-lumen catheter sounds like a good idea, but a second lumen does have a disadvantage in that it increases the diameter of the catheter and the skin puncture site significantly. The two smaller lumens increase the risk of clogging. The vanSonnenberg-D'Agostino gastrojejunal catheter (MediTech) and the Wilms-Oglesby GJ catheter (Cook, Inc.) are single lumen, whereas the Carey-Alzate-Coons GJ catheters (Cook, Inc.) come with either a single or a double lumen (Figs. 3–8 and 3–9). The vanSonnenberg-D'Agostino and Wilms-Oglesby catheters have a mid-catheter loop for gastric retention, whereas the Carey-Alzate-Coons GJ catheters use a Malecot gastric retention device (Figs. 3–8 and 3–9).

Once a tract has been formed successfully over a 2- to 3-week period, some authorities change the G tube for a skin level device. Skin level devices were originally designed for use in pediatric patients because the risk of dislodgment is greatest in babies or children who pull on the G tubes. There are four principal devices available, all consisting of a skin level access port, a valved shaft, and an internal gastric retention mechanism. The Bard Button (Bard Interventional Products, Tewksbury, MA) and the Sandoz Gastroport (Sandoz Nutrition Biosysytems, Minneapolis, MN) have rigid mushrooms for retention (Fig. 3–10). A fluid-filled balloon is used in the MIC-Key (Medical Innovations Corp., Milpetas, CA) and the Wizard (Bard Interventional Products) for gastric retention (Fig. 3–11). The more permanent rigid devices are more difficult to place initially. The balloon devices are more easily placed but necessitate replacement at 6-month intervals due to balloon deflation.

TECHNIQUE MODIFICATIONS

Patients with previous gastric surgery constitute a group in whom percutaneous enteral access can be technically challenging.

Coefficient of Friction

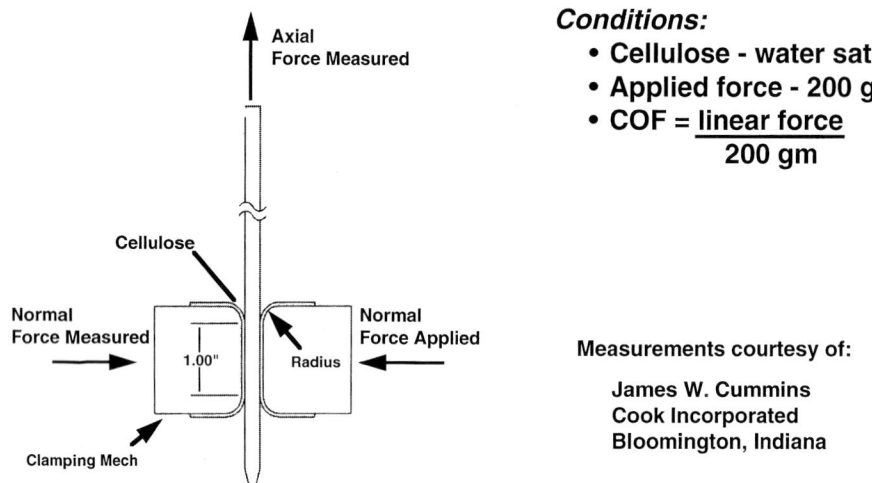

Coefficient of Friction - 86% Reduction

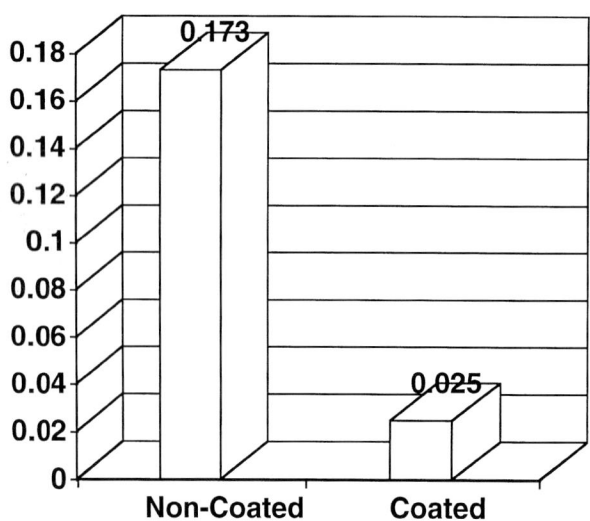

16 Fr Cook Incorporated
ULT-16.0 Ultrathane

Figure 3–7 (A) Apparatus used for the measurement of the coefficient of friction. (B) Graph of the results showing the reduction in coefficient of friction with the hydrophilic coating.

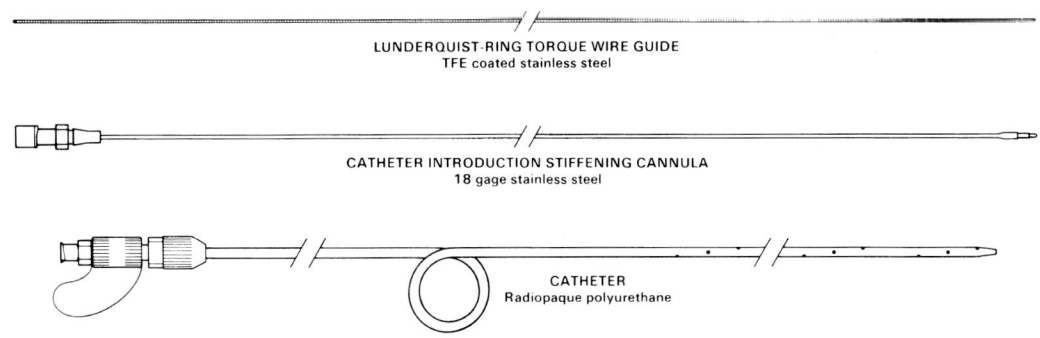

Figure 3–8 The Wilms-Oglesby gastrojejunostomy catheter (Cook, Inc., Bloomington, IN), single lumen.

In patients who have a large enough gastric remnant, a standard technique can be used. The gastric remnant is usually further from the skin surface than the usual site of gastric puncture, necessitating use of a longer puncture needle.[53] Intragastric balloon support has been employed to give better counterforce for the initial gastric puncture.[30,31] In this method, a large balloon is affixed to an NG tube and advanced to the residual gastric lumen or jejunum, if the patient has had a total gastrectomy, and subsequently

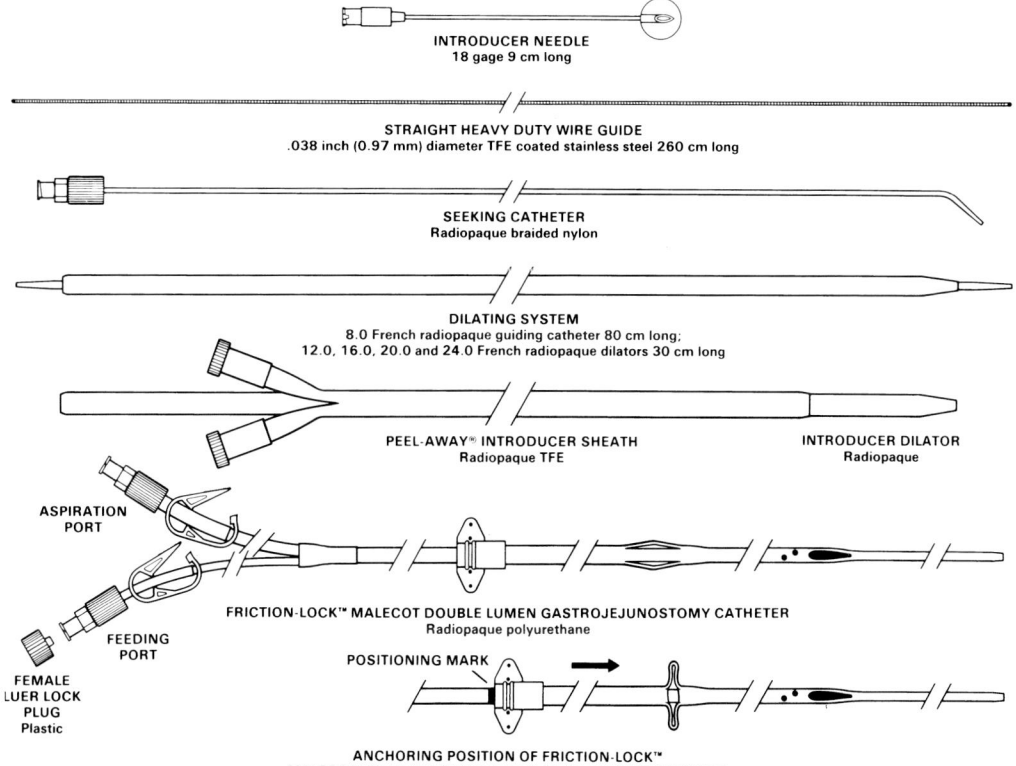

Figure 3–9 The Carey-Alzate-Coons gastrojejunostomy catheters (Cook, Inc., Bloomington, IN), which come in single or double lumen.

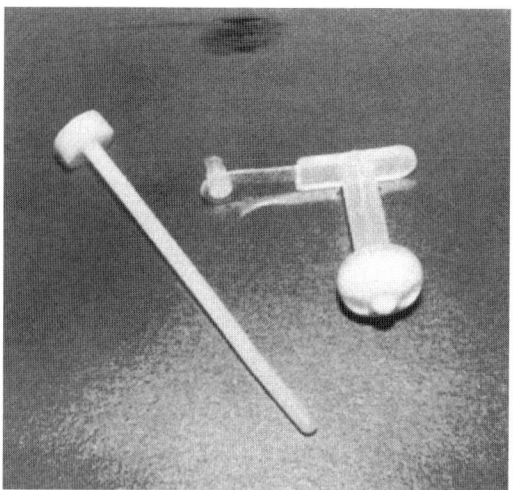

Figure 3–10 The Bard Button with a rigid mushroom bumper.

distended with dilute contrast media. Following inflation of the balloon it is possible to proceed with the percutaneous method as previously with an added degree of confidence with respect to the compliance of the anterior bowel wall.[45] Direct fluoroscopic access using a Chiba needle to a small residual stomach for the purpose of lumen distention is also an option in the postoperative patient.

Another entity that we have encountered, also described in the literature, is an infracolic approach for the placement of percutaneous gastrojejunostomies.[33] In the vast majority of situations, the safer route above the transverse colon is employed. To this end, some clinicians use fluoroscopy or lateral fluoroscopy, and some administer barium prior to the procedure to outline the transverse colon. However, we have noted in very few patients that the transverse colon remains anterior to the ideal gastric puncture site, thus precluding percutaneous placement. In select patients, particularly those who are poor surgical candidates, we have successfully accomplished infracolic gastric access without complication. We have also noted that patients with previous abdominal surgery or patients who have had inadvertent removal of their G tube prior to tract formation more frequently have colon that is anterior to the stomach. This may be due to adhesions or inflammatory response at the gastric puncture site. There is an increased incidence of complications using the infracolic approach to the stomach, specifically hemorrhage. In supracolic gastric puncture, one traverses the anterior abdominal wall, whereas with

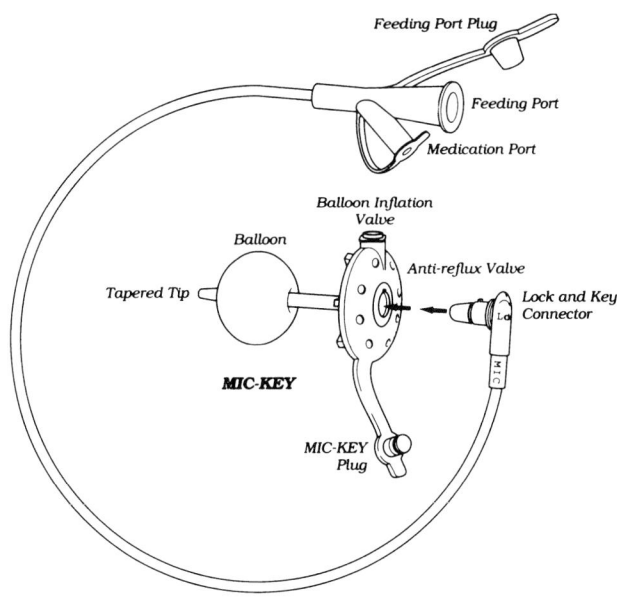

Figure 3–11 The MIC-Key device with a balloon for intragastric retention.

the infracolic approach the greater omentum, transverse mesocolon, gastrocolic ligament, and lesser sac are traversed. Due to the presence of the neurovascular bundle and lymphatics within the transverse mesocolon, which extends from the pancreas to the transverse colon, the increased risk of injury with possible hemorrhage must be carefully considered prior to an attempt at this approach.

Percutaneous Jejunostomy

In situations where percutaneous gastrostomy is difficult, several authorities have described techniques of direct percutaneous jejunostomy as a direct approach to the small bowel. Such techniques are typically carried out in patients who have had previous gastric surgery or resection or extensive tumor infiltration of the gastric wall or whose stomachs lie in a horizontal or difficult-access position. Direct percutaneous jejunostomy has also been done in patients with documented chronic aspiration and in those with gastric outlet obstruction. An unusual indication for this procedure occurs when the patient aspirates persistently despite the presence of a percutaneous endoscopic jejunostomy (PEJ). Initially, PEJ was seen as the procedure of choice in patients with aspiration; however, in recent reports up to 60% of patients with PEJ had persistent aspiration.[54–56] This is most likely secondary to the difficulty that the endoscopist has in advancing the tip of the catheter beyond the ligament of Treitz.[54] Placement of the catheter tip distal to the ligament of Treitz is easier when the percutaneous radiologic technique is used, and with fluoroscopic guidance the operator can be certain of the catheter tip position at the conclusion of the procedure.

The technique for direct percutaneous jejunostomy is similar to that for direct Seldinger gastrostomy. Using lateral fluoroscopic guidance, an NG tube is advanced to the desired level of bowel. One can identify an appropriate loop of jejunum that is close to the skin surface. Alternatively, one can use balloon support as described by Gray et al.[45] The superior epigastric vessels and the rectus abdominal muscles are spared by using a lateral approach in an attempt to directly access the jejunum. Given the tendency of the bowel to move away, a gastropexy device is generally used in direct jejunostomy (Fig. 3–1). We have also used CT in some situations for the initial jejunal access (Fig. 3–2). On access to the jejunum the greater omentum is typically traversed, and one should attempt to puncture the antimesenteric border of the appropriate jejunal loop. The tract is sequentially dilated over a guide wire following placement of a number of gastropexy devices. We tend to use a locking pigtail catheter as our jejunostomy feeding tube and confirm its position by injecting a small volume of contrast agent (Figs. 3–1 and 3–2).

Other techniques have also been described, including combined percutaneous and endoscopic techniques, as described by Westfall et al.[57] The drawbacks of the combined percutaneous and endoscopic technique include the necessity for two physicians, the significant sedation, and the technically demanding methodology. To date, direct percutaneous jejunostomy is not widely performed and the numbers in the literature are small; however, it is a safe and effective alternative to endoscopic or GJ placement in appropriately selected patients.[58]

A newer approach to securing access to the small bowel is percutaneous translumbar duodenostomy.[59,60] The techniques described to date include the use of CT guidance for localization of an appropriate site and tracking to the retroperitoneal duodenum from a translumbar approach. Some authors have used biplane fluoroscopy with an NG tube in the duodenum for appropriate puncture site localization.[50] More recently, a technique involving use of an 8-Fr occlusion-type balloon in the duodenum and appropriate fluoroscopic guidance for puncture has also been described. Until further experience is gained with this particular technique, specific indications and/or contraindications for its use cannot be elucidated.

Results and Complications

Both surgical and endoscopic enteral access techniques have been longer established than radiologic methods. Comparisons between the surgical and endoscopic methods have been published on several occasions,[61-64] but no prospective comparison of nonsurgical methods has been done. However, Wollman et al have done both an institutional evaluation and a meta-analysis of the literature.[41,42]

In comparing the three methods, there are a number of different parameters to be reviewed. First, the procedures must be understood. The surgical technique involves a laparotomy, identification of the midgastric body, and placement of a number of purse-string sutures, followed by a stab incision for the placement of the G tube. A similar stab incision is made in the anterior abdominal wall, and the stomach is sutured to the anterior abdominal wall in an appropriate fashion. More recently, we have seen the introduction of a laparoscopic technique[9,10] that includes the making of the initial gastric puncture with two trochars.

PEG has a number of technical variations. The pull method entails traversing the anterior abdominal wall, withdrawing a suture from the mouth, and using this suture to pull the G tube from the oral cavity to the gastric lumen through the anterior abdominal wall. The push method uses a percutaneous peel-away sheath and advancement of the G tube in that fashion.

When one looks at the three techniques, only in the PEG group does one need to provide some antibiotic prophylaxis; anesthetic requirements vary considerably among the three groups. Both PEG and PG are performed with local anesthesia and varying amounts of intravenous sedation. Wohlman and colleagues in their review report that PG tends to require less sedation than PEG.[40,41]

However, one advantage of PEG placement is that it can be done in the intensive care unit, whereas the surgical technique obviously must be performed in an operating room and PG requires fluoroscopy.

Two operators are required for the performance of a PEG, whereas a single operator can perform either surgical or radiologic gastrostomy. We feel that the time element is a significant advantage of PG over the other two techniques. Our mean procedure time has been 7 minutes, whereas Wollman reports 89 minutes for the surgical gastrostomy and 36 minutes for PEG.[29,40,41]

As physicians who perform procedures on patients, we commonly compare various techniques without taking into consideration patient preference, patient pain, or the level of patient discomfort that is caused by the procedure. With respect to surgical gastrostomy, patients have at least a scar from the G-tube placement, which may be by laparotomy, or laparoscopic incisions with associated postprocedure discomfort. However, the surgical procedure does not entail any transoral manipulation; therefore, the patient is spared this discomfort. With PEG and PG, a degree of oropharyngeal discomfort is present. With PG one passes an NG tube; with PEG one has to pass an endoscope or, in the pull method the G tube, through the oropharynx and esophagus. We must always be aware of the level of discomfort involved, and studies have shown that postprocedure narcotic requirements are significantly lower with PG than with PEG or surgical gastrostomy.[40,41]

Surgical series have a 100% technical success rate. Even in cases where an occult malignancy is identified, a jejunostomy can commonly be fashioned. In most series, PGs have a higher technical success rate than PEGs.[65-69]

A commonly quoted advantage of PEG is that additional diagnostic information can be yielded by endoscopy. However, Wollman's institutional review showed that none of the additional clinical findings noted at endoscopy made alteration in patient management necessary or indicated that G-tube placement was required.

Surgical gastrostomy had the highest overall complication rate (29%) and the highest major complication rate (19.9%) of the three procedures. There was no significant difference in overall complication rates between radiologic and PEG percutaneous techniques, whereas tube-related complications were fewer in those placed by radiologists.[40,41]

In PG, initial fluoroscopy and choice of appropriate access site and path are critical. A number of authors use preprocedure ultrasonography to identify the liver and/or oral contrast media administered on the day prior to outline the transverse colon. We depend largely on fluoroscopic guidance. Most of the intra-abominal organs have been punctured on occasion, including small and large bowel and liver. When identified quickly, such complications usually can be dealt with without resorting to surgery. Small bowel injury in general does not need any specific therapy other than careful monitoring, whereas a colonic, or most commonly transcolonic, injury can be managed as a controlled fistula. Traversing the liver is not the ideal approach, but because we traverse this organ regularly for other interventional procedures, transhepatic G-tube placement may not be a significant problem. Obviously, when one performs the procedure surgically the transgression of nontarget organs should not happen, but this has been described after PEG with subsequent enteral cutaneous fistulae.[70,71] With respect to wound and puncture site problems, the PEG procedure has an increased risk of infection, which is decreased by the use of prophylactic antibiotics. In a well-structured study by Akkersdijk et al,[72] the pull method with and without antibiotics was performed. There was a decrease in periaccess site infection from 41% to 14% with the use of prophylactic antibiotics; however, this rate was decreased to zero when both prophylactic antibiotics and the push method were used. With respect to hemorrhagic complications, the number of punctures and sites of gastrostomy are particularly important. Again, we puncture the standard midanterior wall of the stomach because this is a relatively avascular plane, and we have had no major bleeding problems. We also correct any coagulopathies prior to gastrostomy placement.

In the early postprocedure period, the potential for peritonitis to develop (incidence of less than 1%) is a significant worry and one that remains debatable with respect to the methods for decreasing its incidence. Early displacement of tubes and other tube-related complications are most worrisome during the first week, when there has been insufficient time for proper tract formation. Once the tract has matured, it is relatively easy to replace the catheter over a guide wire with fluoroscopic guidance. However, tract disruption in the first 7 days is a leading cause of repeated procedures. If the catheter becomes dislodged during that early period, we recommend NG suction, bowel rest for 48 hours, and a fresh attempt at gastrostomy. One advantage of gastropexy becomes relevant in the case of early catheter dislodgment because the presence of the gastropexy device makes replacement relatively easy. In a geriatric patient with Parkinson's disease in whom we placed a G tube for nutritional support, a second placement resulted in a transcolonic placement (Fig. 3–12). We have noted that extra care must be taken in patients with any previous abdominal violation due to the anatomical changes that are commonly present. The second point illustrated in this case is that in patients who are at risk of removing or pulling on the G tube, an abdominal binder of some kind is essential for the first week at least. We do not feel that reports in the literature prove the global benefit of gastropexy; therefore, it is not part of our standard technique. However, we are more liberal in our use of gastropexy devices in these patients to facilitate easier and less risky replacements. If a partial displacement is reported, early fluoroscopy, contrast examination, and

CHAPTER 3 · PERCUTANEOUS GASTROSTOMY, GASTROENTEROSTOMY, AND JEJUNOSTOMY

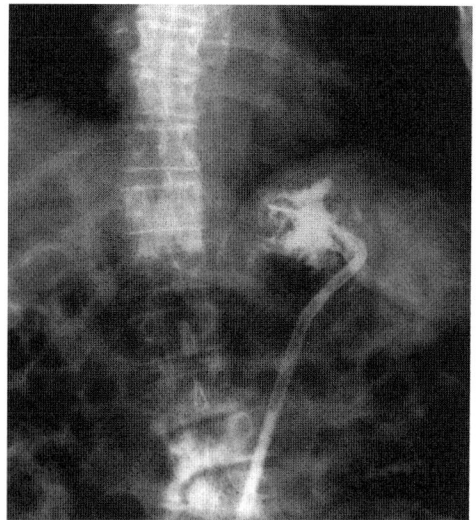

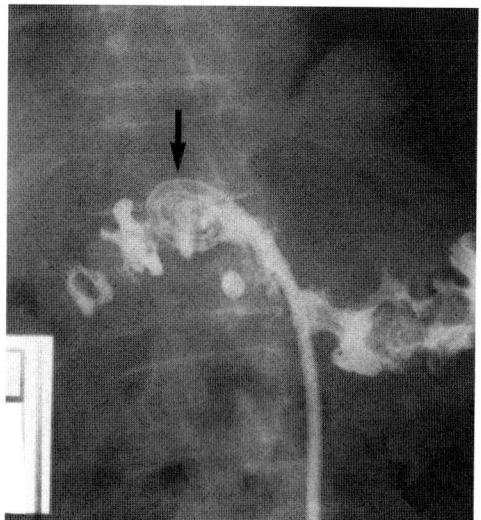

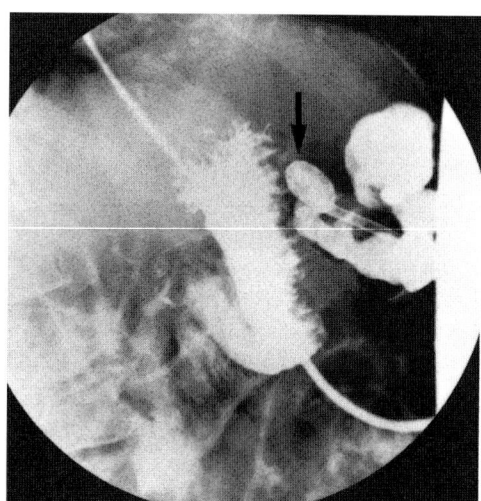

Figure 3–12 An 83-year-old man with end-stage Parkinson's disease in need of gastrostomy tube for nutritional support. **(A)** Initial fluoroscopic image post initial uncomplicated G-tube placement with contrast injection confirming intragastric positioning. **(B)** Two weeks later, after patient was noted to be tugging on catheter and having some diarrhea. Contrast examination of the G tube confirms the catheter loop to be in the transverse colon (*arrow*). **(C)** A further study on the following day via a nass gastric tube demonstrates no leak from the gastric puncture site and the G-tube remaining in the colon (*arrow*).

repositioning or replacement is indicated. We urge that this be done as early as possible because the tract can close surprisingly quickly (Fig. 3–13).

Once the catheter is in place it can also be displaced within the gastrointestinal tract (Figs. 3–14 to 3–17). The distal end of the G tube may be displaced and present significant clinical problems. We have seen the solid bumper of a PEG tube advance to the pylorus, resulting in pyloric obstruction (Fig. 3–14). If the catheter is balloon-tipped, the balloon can advance with peristalsis, resulting in small bowel obstruction, or it can act as the lead point for intussusception (Figs. 3–15 and 3–16). In these situations when the patient complains of new obstruction or discomfort, early fluoroscopic contrast examination is usually diagnostic. Catheter manipulation and/or re-placement is typically curative at the same sitting.

Most common problems and complications are related to clogging or accidental removal of the catheter. Tube clogging can and should be avoided if attention is paid

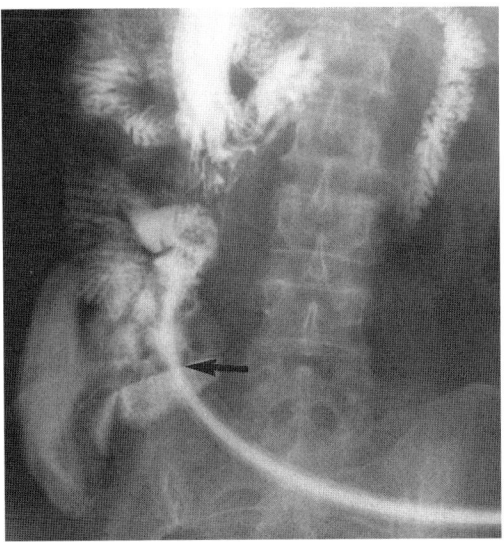

Figure 3–13 Patient complained of excessive site leakage. Contrast study shows G tube partially withdrawn along the tract (*arrow*). Catheter was easily advanced and repositioned, resulting in resolution of symptoms.

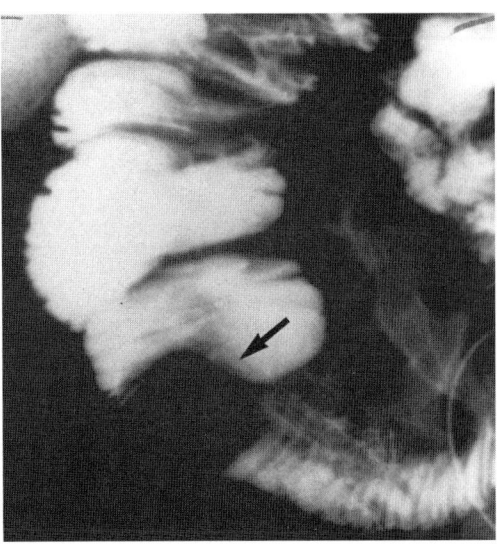

Figure 3–15 Balloon-tipped G tube has migrated to the distal duodenum and caused partial small bowel obstruction (*arrow*).

to catheter maintenance. Using only liquid feeds and medications and vigorous flushing after each use is the order of the day. If the catheter gets clogged, high-pressure

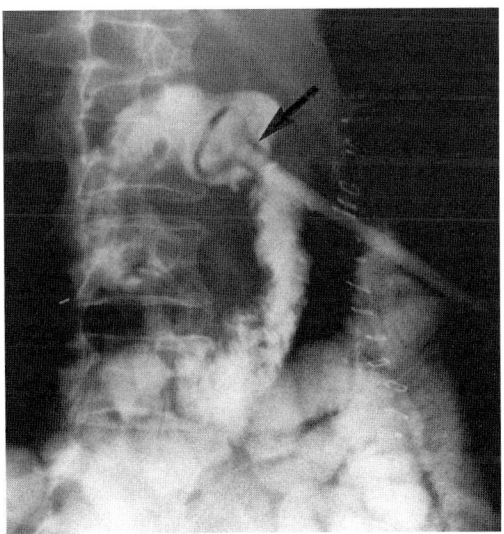

Figure 3–14 Rigid bumper of a percutaneous endoscopic gastrostomy tube that has migrated to the pyloric canal, causing partial pyloric obstruction (*arrow*).

vigorous injection (1-cm^3 syringe) or injection of carbonated liquids will solve the problem. We have on occasion resorted to the use of a glide wire (MediTech) to open a channel in resistant cases.

Site erythema and infection are relatively common occurrences (4%). Local therapy with frequent dressing changes and cleaning may suffice. We have used peroxide washes for short periods with local discharges to prevent local infection. If frank infection (pus or abscess) is present, then more aggressive management with antibiotics and wound care is appropriate.

SUMMARY

Percutaneous gastrostomy is a valuable technique with proven advantages over surgical gastrostomy. Recently, radiologic percutaneous gastrostomy has been demonstrated to have some advantage over endoscopic techniques with respect to complication rates and technical success.[25,40] As attested to in a recent paper by Bell et al, the major and minor complication rates of 1.3% and 2.9%,

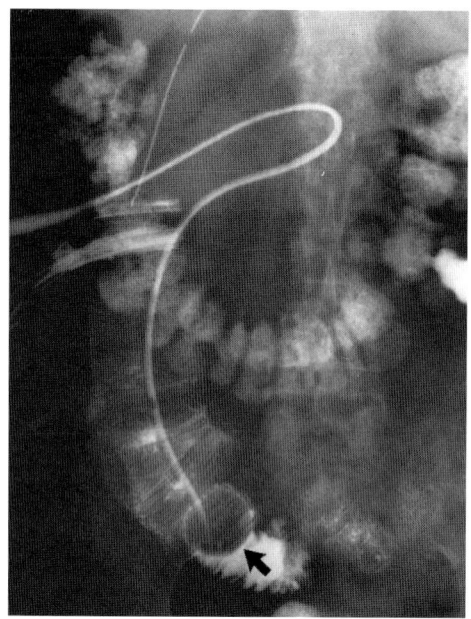 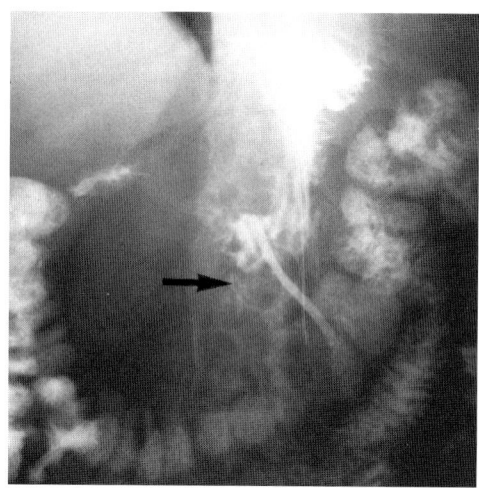

Figure 3–16 (A) A balloon-tipped G tube has migrated to the jejunum and acted as lead point for an intussusception (*arrow*). (B) Post fluoroscopy-guided withdrawal of catheter. The balloon is now in good position (*arrow*).

respectively, are attractive and should encourage radiologists to offer and perform this procedure more frequently.[25]

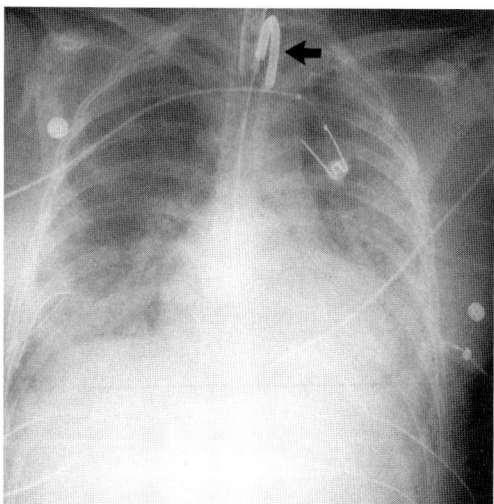

Figure 3–17 Patient with a large-bore surgical G tube in place and endoscopic attempt at trans-G-tube/J-tube placement. Tip of the jejunal feeding tube is coiled in the pharynx (*arrow*).

References

1. Moore JP, Curreri PW, Rodning CB. Percutaneous endoscopic gastrostomy. *Am Surg* 1986;52(9):495–499.
2. Gauderer MW, Stellato TA. Gastrostomies: evolution, techniques, indications, and complications. *Curr Probl Surg* 1986;23:657–719.
3. Egeberg CA. Om behandlingen af impenetrable stricturer I madr'ret (oesophagus). *Norsk Mag Laegevidensk* 1841;2:97–106.
4. Walker LG, Staton LL. The first successful gastrostomy in America. *Surg Gynecol Obstet* 1984;158:387–388.
5. Gauderer MWL, Ponsky JL, Izant RJ. Gastrostomy without laparotomy: a percutaneous endoscopic technique. *J Pediatr Surg* 1980;15:872–875.
6. Ponsky JL. Percutaneous endoscopic gastrostomy: review of 150 cases. *Arch Surg* 1983 Aug;118:913–914.
7. Preshaw RM. A percutaneous method for inserting a feeding gastrostomy tube. *Surg Gynecol Obstet* 1981;152:659–660.
8. Torosian MH, Rombeau JL. Feeding by tube enterostomy. *Surg Gynecol Obstet* 1980;150:918–924.

9. Edelman DS, Unger SW. Laparoscopic gastrostomy. *Surg Gynecol Obstet* 1991;173:401.
10. Duh Q-Y, Way LW. Laparoscopic jejunostomy using T-fasteners as retractors and anchors. *Arch Surg* 1993 Jan;128:105–108.
11. Sachs BA, Gotzer DK. Percutaneous re-establishment of feeding gastrostomies. *Surgery* 1979;85:576–577.
12. Russell TR, Brotman M, Norris F. Percutaneous gastrostomy: a new simplified and cost-effective technique. *Am J Surg* 1984 Jul;148:132–137.
13. Norton B, Homer-Ward M, Donnelly MT, Long RG, Holmes GK. A randomised prospective comparison of percutaneous endoscopic gastrostomy and nasogastric tube feeding after acute dysphagic stroke. *BMJ* 1996;312:13–16.
14. Park RHR, Allison MC, Lang J, et al. Randomized comparison of percutaneous endoscopic gastrostomy and naso-gastric tube feeding in patients with persisting neurological dysphagia. *BMJ* 1992;304: 1406–1409.
15. Baskin WN. Advances in enteral nutrition techniques. *Am J Gastroenterol* 1992;87(11): 1547–1553.
16. Bistrian BR, Blackburn GL, Vitale J, et al. Prevalence of malnutrition in general medical patients. *JAMA* 1976;235:1567–1570.
17. Burtch GD, Shatney CH. Feeding jejunostomy (versus gastrostomy) passes the test of time. *Am Surg* 1987;53:54–57.
18. Souba WW. The gut as a nitrogen-processing organ in the metabolic response to critical illness. *Nutr Sup Serv* 1988;8:15–22.
19. Alverdy J, Chi HS, Sheldon GF. The effect of parenteral nutrition on gastrointestinal immunity: the importance of enteral stimulation. *Ann Surg* 1985;202:681–684.
20. Daly JM, Lieberman M, Goldfine J, et al. Enteral nutrition with supplemental arginine, RNA and omega-3 fatty acids: a prospective clinical trial. *J Parent Ent Nutr* 1991;15:19S.
21. Waitzberg DL, Braz E, Gama-Rodrigues J, et al. Postoperative enteral nutrition support in complicated cardiac surgery. *Nutr Clin Pract* 1986;1:250–266.
22. Cabre E, Gonzalez-Huix F, Abad-Lacruz A, et al. Effect of total enteral nutrition on the short-term outcome of severely malnourished cirrhotics. *Gastroenterology* 1990;98: 715–720.
23. O'Keefe F, Carrasco CH, Charnsangavej C, et al. Percutaneous drainage and feeding gastrostomies in 100 patients. *Radiology* 1989;172:341–343.
24. Ryan JM, Hahn PF, Boland GW, McDowell RK, Saini S, Mueller PR. Percutaneous gastrostomy with T-fastener gastropexy: results of 316 consecutive procedures. *Radiology* 1997;203:496–500.
25. Bell SD, Carmody EA, Yeung EY, Thurston WA, Simons ME, Ho C-S. Percutaneous gastrostomy and gastrojejunostomy: additional experience in 519 procedures. *Radiology* 1995;194:817–820.
26. Olson DL, Krubsack AJ, Stewart ET. Percutaneous enteral alimentation: gastrostomy versus gastrojejunostomy. *Radiology* 1993; 187:105–108.
27. Gustke RF, Varma RR, Soergel KH. Gastric reflux during perfusion of the proximal small bowel. *Gastroenterology* 1970;59:890–895.
28. Lazarus BA, Murphy JB, Culpepper L. Aspiration associated with long-term gastric versus jejunal feeding: a critical analysis of the literature. *Arch Phys Med Rehabil* 1990; 71:46–52.
29. Deutsch LS, Kannegieter L, Vanson DT, Miller DP, Brandon JC. Simplified percutaneous gastrostomy. *Radiology* 1992;184:181–183.
30. Varney RA, vanSonnenberg E, Giovanna C, Sukthankar R. Balloon techniques for percutaneous gastrostomy in a patient with partial gastrectomy. *Radiology* 1988;167:69–70.
31. vanSonnenberg E, Cubberley A, Brown K, et al. Percutaneous gastrostomy: use of intragastric balloon. *Radiology* 1984;152:531–532.
32. Kanazawa S, Naomoto Y, Yasui K, Kato K, Nakamura K, Hiraki Y. Percutaneous transhepatic feeding gastrostomy performed with CT guidance in patients with partial gastrectomy (Abstr). *Radiology* 1993;189(P):337.
33. Mirich DR, Gray RR. Infracolic percutaneous gastrojejunostomy: technical note. *Cardiovasc Intervent Radiol* 1990;12:340–341.
34. Shellito PC, Malt RA. Tube gastrostomy: technique and complications. *Ann Surg* 1985; 201:180–195.
35. Ho C-S. Percutaneous gastrostomy for jejunal feeding. *Radiology* 1983;149:595–596.
36. Wills JS, Oglesby T. Percutaneous gastrostomy. *Radiology* 1983;149:449–453.
37. Alzate GD, Coons HG, Elliot J, Carey PH. Percutaneous gastrostomy for jejunal

feeding: a new technique. *Am J Roentgenol* 1986;147:822-825.
38. Halkier BK, Ho C-S, Yee ACN. Percutaneous feeding gastrostomy with the Seldinger technique: review of 252 patients. *Radiology* 1989; 171:359–362.
39. Saini S, Mueller PR, Gaa J, et al. Percutaneous gastrostomy with gastropexy: experience in 125 patients. *Am J Roentgenol* 1990; 154: 1003–1006.
40. Ho C-S, Yeung EY. Percutaneous gastrostomy and transgastric jejunostomy. *Am J Roentgenol* 1992;158:0251–0257.
41. Wollman B, D'Agostino HB, Walus-Wigle JR, Easter DW, Beale A. Radiologic, endoscopic, and surgical gastrostomy: an institutional evaluation and meta-analysis of the literature. *Radiology* 1995;197:699–704.
42. Wollman B, D'Agostino HB, Walus-Wigle JR, et al. Radiologic, endoscopic and surgical gastrostomy: an institutional review and meta-analysis of the literature. *Clin Radiol* 1996;51:820–822.
43. Chait PG, Weinberg J, Connolly BL, et al. Retrograde percutaneous gastrostomy and gastrojejunostomy in 505 children: a 4 1/2-year experience. *Radiology* 1996;201:691–695.
44. Cope C. Suture anchor for visceral drainage. *Am J Roentgenol* 1986;146:160–161.
45. Gray RR, Ho CS, Yee A, Montanera W, Jones DP. Direct percutaneous jejunostomy. *Am J Roentgenol* 1987;149:931–932.
46. Light VL, Slezak FA, Porter JA, Gerson LW, McCord G. Predictive factors for early mortality after percutaneous endoscopic gastrostomy. *Gastointest Endosc* 1995;42:330–335.
47. Marx MV, William DM, Perkins AJ, et al. Percutaneous feeding tube placement in pediatric patients: immediate and 30-day results. *J Vasc Intervent Radiol* 1996;7:107–115.
48. Marx MV, Andrews JC. Conversion of gastrostomy tube to gastrojejunostomy tube. *Am J Roentgenol* 1993;161:902–903.
49. Lu DSK, Mueller PR, Lee MJ, Dawson SL, Hahn PF, Brountzos E. Gastrostomy conversion to transgastric jejunostomy: technical problems, causes of failure, and proposed solutions in 63 patients. *Radiology* 1993;187: 679–683.
50. Kerns SR. Conversion of gastrostomy tube to gastrojejunostomy tube by using a peel-away sheath. *Am J Roentgenol* 1993;160: 206–207.
51. Bender GN, Haggerty MF. A third technique for converting a gastrostomy tube to a gastrojejunostomy tube. *Am J Roentgenol* 1994; 162:1501.
52. Burdick JS, Venu R, Hogan W. Replacement of the percutaneous gastrostomy tube: is the indirect non-endoscopic visualization technique safe? *Gastrointest Endosc* 1993;39:A249.
53. Stevens S, Picus D, Hicks ME, Darcy MD, Vesely TM, Kleinhoffer MA. Percutaneous gstrostomy and gastrojejunostomy after gastric surgery. *J Vasc Intervent Radiol* 1992;3: 679–683.
54. DiSario JA, Foutch PG, Sanowski RA. Poor results with percutaneous endoscopic jejunostomy. *Gastrointest Endosc* 1990;36:257–260.
55. Wolfsen HC, Kozarek RA, Ball TJ, Patterson DJ, Botoman VA. Tube dysfunction following percutaneous endoscopic gastrostomy and jejunostomy. *Gastrointest Endosc* 1990;36: 261–263.
56. Kadakia SC, Sullivan HO, Starnes E. Percutaneous endoscopic gastrostomy or jejunostomy and the incidence of aspiration in 79 patients. *Am J Surg* 1992;164:114–118.
57. Westfall SH, Andrews CH, Naunheim KS. A reproducible, safe jejunostomy replacement technique by a percutaneous endoscopic method. *Am Surg* 1990;56:141–143.
58. Hallisey MJ, Pollard JC. Direct percutaneous jejunostomy. *J Vasc Intervent Radiol* 1994;5: 625–632.
59. Koolpe HA, Dorfman D, Kramer M. Translumbar duodenostomy for enteral feeding. *Am J Roentgenol* 1989;153:299–300.
60. Cwikiel W. Percutaneous duodenostomy—alternative route for enteral nutrition. *Acta Radiologica* 1991;32:153–154.
61. Davis JB Jr, Bowden TA Jr, Rives DA. Percutaneous endoscopic gastrostomy: do surgeons and gastroenterologists get the same results? *Am Surg* 1990;56:47–51.
62. Stiegmann GV, Goff JS, Silas D, Pearlman N, Sun J, Norton L. Endoscopic versus operative gastrostomy: final results of a prospective randomized trial. *Gastrointest Endosc* 1990;36(1):1–5.
63. Jones M, Santanello SA, Falcone RE. Percutaneous endoscopic vs. surgical gastrostomy. *J Parent Ent Nutr* 1990;14(5):533–534.
64. Elliott LA, Sheridan MB, Denyer M, Chapman AH. PEG—is the E necessary? A comparison of percutaneous and endoscopic gastrostomy. *Clin Radiol* 1996;51:341–344.

65. Au FC. The Stamm gastrostomy: a sound procedure. *Am Surg* 1993;59:674–675.
66. Wasiljew B, Ujiki G, Beal J. Feeding gastrostomy: complications and mortality. *Am J Surg* 1982;143:194–195.
67. Ruge J, Vasques RM. An analysis of the advantage of the Stamm and percutaneous gastrostomy. *Surg Gynecol Obstet* 1986;162:13–16.
68. Albanase CT, Towbin RB, Ulman I, Lewis J, Smith SD. Percutaneous gastrojejunostomy versus Nissen fundoplication for enteral feeding of the neurologically impaired child with gastroesophageal reflux. *J Pediatr* 1993;123:371–375.
69. Hicks ME, Surratt RS, Picus D, Marx MV, Lang EV. Fluoroscopically guided percutaneous gastrostomy and gastroenterostomy: analysis of 158 consecutive cases. *Am J Roentgenol* 1990;154:725–728.
70. Marin OE, Glassman MS, Schoen BT, Caplan DB. Safety and efficacy of percutaneous endoscopic gastrostomy in children. *Am J Gastroenterol* 1994;89:359–362.
71. Scapa E, Broide E, Slutzi S, Halevy A. Colocutaneous fistula—a rare complication of percutaneous endoscopic gastrostomy. *Surg Laparosc Endosc* 1993;3:430–432.
72. Akkersdijk WL, van Bergeijk JD, van Egmond T, et al. Percutaneous endoscopic gastrostomy (PEG): comparison of push and pull methods and evaluation of antibiotic prophylactics. *Endoscopy* 1995;27:313–316.

Chapter 4

Percutaneous Colostomy

Lorenzo Carson
Elvira Lang

Decompression of distal bowel obstruction has traditionally belonged in the surgical domain. Although surgical colostomy is generally considered to be a safe procedure, poor patient health may make even this intervention prohibitively risky. In such cases, percutaneous techniques provide a less invasive alternative. In 1985, Crass et al described computed tomography (CT)–guided percutaneous needle aspiration of cecal gas from a massively distended cecum in Ogilvie's syndrome.[1] Since then, several modifications of the percutaneous technique have been introduced to reduce the potential for peritoneal spillage and to improve drainage and decompression. Indications for percutaneous colostomy are still evolving, and optimal approaches are not yet defined. For the majority of applications, experience is anecdotal. We compiled the limited information available on percutaneous colostomy to provide a guide for decision making regarding this relatively new realm of intervention. The following sections will identify current indications, technical considerations, and potential pitfalls of percutaneous colostomy.

INDICATIONS

Percutaneous colostomy has been used for the following indications:

- Cecal decompression
- Ogilvie's syndrome
- Detorsion of cecal volvulus
- Colonic irrigation for treatment of fecal incontinence
- Colonic irrigation with antibiotics
- Draining enterostomy
- Management of intestinal gas lock

Cecal Decompression and Ogilvie's Syndrome

Massive and prolonged distention of the cecum to diameters of 10 to 12 cm or greater has been associated with an increased risk of perforation.[2,3] Perforation can be expected in up to 25% of cases.[3,4] The risk of perforation correlates more strongly with the duration of cecal distention than the absolute diameter.[2,4] When perforation occurs, mortality reaches 43 to 46%.[2,3] Common causes of cecal distention include mechanical colonic obstruction and so-called pseudo-obstruction (Ogilvie's syndrome). Cecal volvulus is responsible for 0.8 to 4.1% of cases of intestinal obstruction.[5,6]

Ogilvie in 1948,[7] and Dunlop shortly thereafter,[8] described three patients with recurrent clinical signs of large bowel obstruction in the absence of organic stenoses. Both authors noted that passing flatus brought relief. These first reported patients had malignant infiltration of their sympathetic or parasympathetic nerve chains, and a disturbance of colonic innervation with parasympathetic overreaction was assumed to cause the colonic spasm. However, autopsy studies failed to reveal inherent abnormalities of the colon or nerve chains of subsequent patients with intestinal pseudo-obstruction.[9] Intestinal pseudo-obstruction can be encountered at any age but is most common in the sixth decade.[2,3] Associated conditions are common (93%) and include preceding abdominal, obstetrical, or orthopedic surgery, thoracic or cardiovascular operations, trauma, myocardial infarction, and neurologic diseases.[3,10] Urologic surgery is the most common associated condition in men and the second most common in women.[3]

Ogilvie's syndrome is characterized by massive colonic dilatation in the absence of organic obstruction. This dilatation is most commonly segmental, involving the cecum and the ascending and transverse colon, but can reach the rectosigmoid.[2] The cecum is the most common site of perforation. According to Laplace's law, the wall tension of a hollow viscus is proportional to its diameter for a given intraluminal pressure. Increasing wall tension leads to gradual reduction and cessation of capillary, venous, and, finally, arterial flow.[11] The combination of increased intraluminal pressure and ischemic impairment of the bowel wall facilitates perforation. If the intestine is decompressed and microcirculatory perfusion is restored, no serious sequelae ensue.

Despite the potential self-limiting characteristics, the overall mortality in Ogilvie's may reach 32% even when appropriate therapy is initiated.[9] Supportive care, nasogastric suction, and colonoscopic decompression are considered the initial modes of treatment. Initial colonoscopic decompression is successful in 81% of cases and can serve as definitive treatment in 64 to 86%.[9,10,12] However, the rate of perforation and mortality is not negligible with colonoscopic decompression.[9] Surgical tube colos-tomy has been reserved for endoscopic failures but also has a high mortality. It is in this setting that percutaneous approaches were first described.[1,13] Crass et al[1] used a posterior access to the ascending colon with a 22-gauge Chiba needle under CT guidance and manually aspirated 1500 cm^3 gas from a patient with a 10-cm dilated cecum in whom other treatment modes had failed. Immediate decompression was noted and recovery ensued. Casola et al[13] and vanSonnenberg et al[14] obtained successful decompression in several cases with 5- to 12-Fr catheters. Based on experience gained from managing a patient with Ogilvie's symptomatology, we speculate that colonic air locks can cause Ogilvie's syndrome, thereby affecting treatment options (see below).

Colonic Irrigation for Treatment of Fecal Incontinence

Patients with spina bifida and those having been subjected to trauma or operative procedures on the anus, rectum, or spine can lose normal function of the internal and/or external anal sphincter (Fig. 4–1). Severe constipation and secondary involuntary passage of feces may result and greatly impair lifestyle. Patients with cystic fibrosis are also at risk of developing constipation due to the highly viscous intestinal content (Fig. 4–2). Shandling and others[15] used antegrade irrigation of the colon through a percutaneous cecostomy and inflatable retention balloons in the anal canal to produce controlled evacuations in a larger series of children with encopresis. The percutaneous cecostomy provides access for controlled enemas several times per week, preventing defecation accidents.[15,16]

Colonic Irrigation with Antibiotics

Haaga et al[17] presented a case report of a 67-year-old woman who developed pseudomembranous colitis as a result of intermittent use of oral antibiotics for an infected sinus tract. The patient had been unsuccessfully treated with intravenous metronidazole and vancomycin by nasogastric tube and enema. A retroperitoneal cecostomy was placed using a 5-Fr pigtail catheter, under CT guidance, to provide direct vancomycin instillation into the lumen of the colon. The patient did not improve,

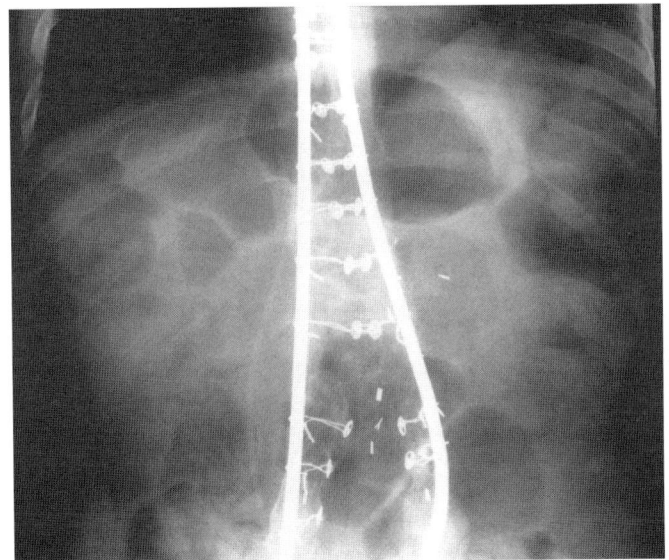

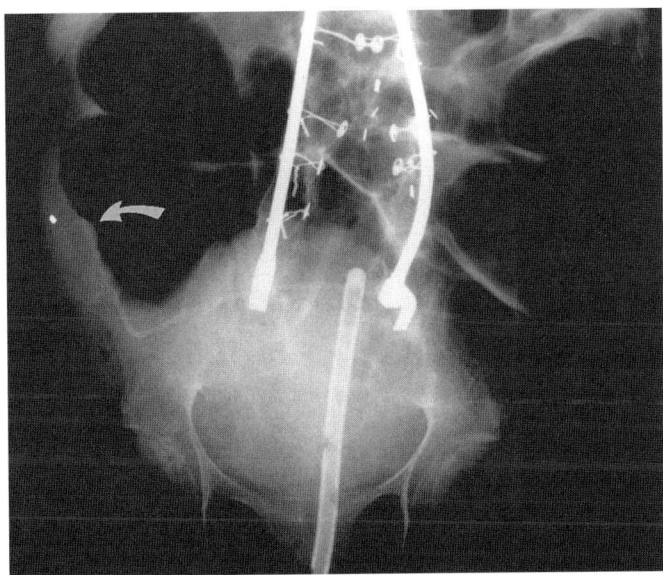

Figure 4–1 20-year-old male patient with meningomyelocele who suffered from severe constipation following spinal fusion. Tube placement (*arrow*) for colonic irrigation. **(A)** Before and **(B)** after tube colostomy. (Courtesy of Dr. S. Kao, University of Iowa Hospital and Clinics).

and a subtotal colectomy with ileostomy was performed. Examination of the resected specimen revealed no evidence of leak at the cecostomy site. Due to lack of clinical trials, this therapy currently has limited application. However, the potential for therapeutic benefit may exist under the right clinical conditions.

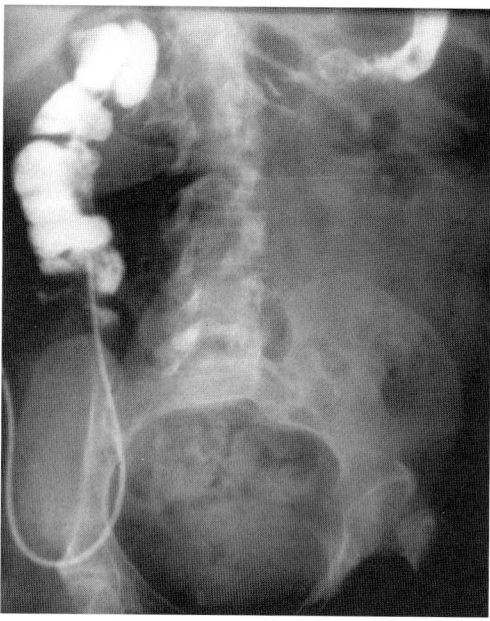

Figure 4–2 Tube colostomy for colonic irrigation in a 24-year-old patient with cystic fibrosis. (Courtesy of Dr. S. Kao, University of Iowa Hospital and Clinics.)

Cecostomy for Detorsion of Cecal Volvulus

Volvulus of the cecum is responsible for 0.8 to 4.1% of cases of intestinal obstruction, with surgery being the treatment of choice.[5,6] Surgical approaches include tube cecostomy or appendicostomy with fixation of the cecum to the lateral abdominal wall or retroperitoneum, if the bowel is viable, and exteriorization with double-barrel enterostomy or right hemicolectomy, if the bowel is not viable.[5] Patel et al[18] used percutaneous anterior transperitoneal decompression of a cecal volvulus in a poor-risk surgical patient. This patient had a history of severe chronic obstructive lung disease. The anterior location of a dilated cecum abutting the anterior abdominal wall was confirmed with a cross-table lateral radiograph. A 16-gauge intracatheter needle was introduced into the dilated cecum, with immediate decompression and detorsion of the cecal volvulus. The needle was withdrawn after fecal occlusion occurred. A small pneumoperitoneum was noted, and follow-up barium enema outlined a normal cecum. Patel believed that puncture of distended cecum is not analogous to inadvertent puncture of bowel loops. Broad-spectrum antibiotics were not considered mandatory. The patient was discharged 4 days after the procedure.

When considering cecostomy for detorsion of cecal volvulus the operator is advised to assure viability of the intestine. There may also be a theoretical advantage to placing a tube cecostomy rather than doing a simple one-step decompression. A tube tract may provide a mechanism of "fixation" that could prevent future episodes of cecal volvulus. It is important that tube cecostomy is not performed after perforation takes place. Perforation is considered to be a surgical emergency (Fig. 4–3).

Draining Enterostomy

Surgical colostomy has remained the treatment of choice for mechanical bowel obstruction. Experience with percutaneous tube colostomy for the treatment of mechanical bowel obstruction is limited. Drainage enterostomies require the use of large-bore tubes for evacuation of feces. Morrison et al[19] percutaneously placed a 24-Fr catheter into the cecum for decompression and palliative drainage in a 71-year-old patient with end-stage cervical carcinoma and distal bowel obstruction. The same authors also performed a successful transperitoneal percutaneous cecostomy and drained approximately 5 L of fluid stool in an 80-year-old patient with an obstruction at the level of the transverse colon.

Percutaneous drainage of intestinal content from an obstructed system bears a considerable risk of pericatheter leakage[20,21] and requires special attention to technical matters (see below). An attractive alternative for patients with mechanical bowel obstruction is transrectal placement of self-expanding metallic stents; this procedure permits rapid resolution of obstruction and subsequent single-stage surgical reconstruction.[22,23]

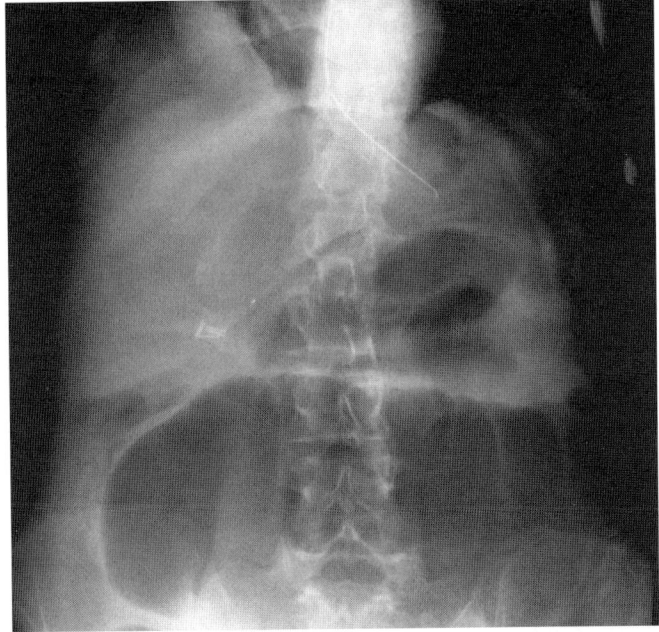

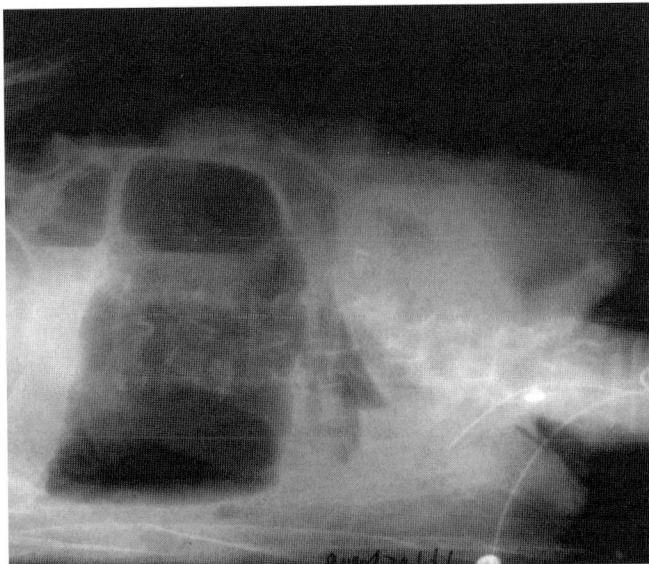

Figure 4–3 Perforated cecal volvulus. **(A)** supine and **(B)** lateral decubitus film. Note large amount of free air.

CHAPTER 4 · PERCUTANEOUS COLOSTOMY

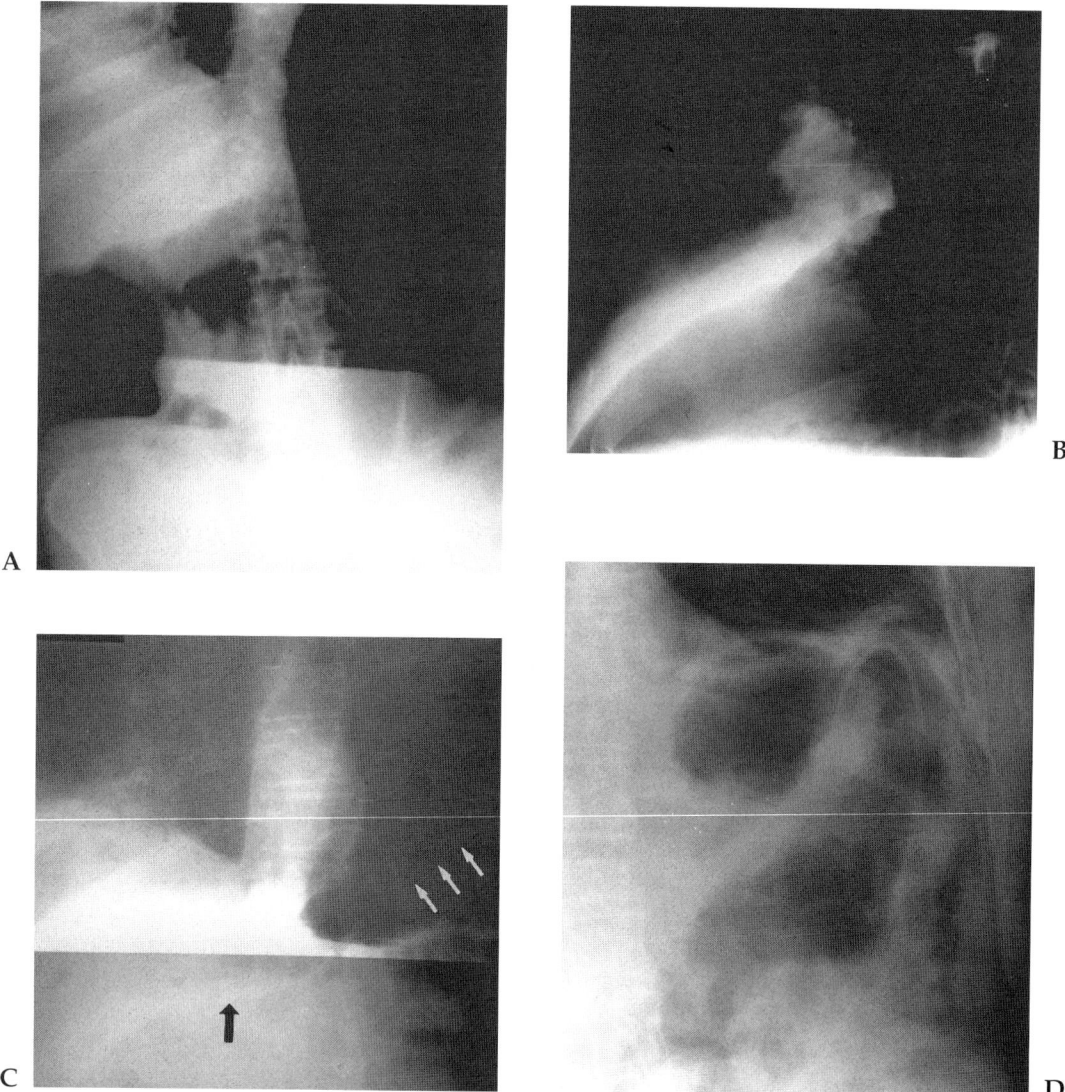

Figure 4–4 A 66-year-old man with amyotrophic lateral sclerosis presented with massive colonic distention extending to the splenic flexure. **(A)** Anteroposterior projection showing massive air-fluid level. To permit visualization of air-containing components and soft tissue, a composite photograph with different exposures was obtained (glued at vertical transition line). **(B)** Lateral projection. Note inverted-U configuration of relatively undistended splenic flexure. **(C)** Note residual air in the splenic flexure after decompression through large-bore drain (*black arrow*). Placement of 7-Fr pigtail catheter (*white arrows*) into the splenic flexure. **(D)** Long-term management with daily gas aspirations from the 7-Fr catheter in the splenic flexure.

Management of Intestinal Gas Locks

We had the opportunity to treat a 66-year-old patient with amyotrophic lateral sclerosis who developed acute exacerbation of chronic colonic distention. This wheelchair-confined man developed immediate hypoxemia in the recumbent position. Given the high risk of ventilator dependency of this patient, the surgical team decided that percutaneous colostomy was the procedure of choice (Fig. 4–4).

The patient was treated sitting on the raised footboard of a fluoroscopy tilt-table. Preprocedure antibiotics and intravenous fentanyl were given prior to fluoroscopic localization of a distended transverse colon. An 18-gauge needle was introduced using an anterior approach following local anesthesia with 1% lidocaine. A single T tack was also introduced to secure the bowel to the anterior abdominal wall. A one-step dilatation set (radial expanding dilator) was used to provide a 12-Fr tube access, which led to immediate decompression of the highly pressurized intestinal contents. A 12-Fr tube, and subsequently 24- and 30-Fr tubes, was used to drain intestinal content. After initial improvement and despite tube patency, the patient developed recurrent bouts of colonic distention that were attributed to formation of a gas lock at the splenic flexure. The patient was subsequently managed with a 7-Fr pigtail catheter placed in the left colonic flexure. With daily aspirations of 150 to 300 mL gas from the splenic flexure he was able to evacuate stool from the rectum and remained nondistended until his death approximately 17 months later. He succumbed to an epidural hematoma after a fall from his wheelchair.

Colonic gas locks can be seen in analogy to accumulation of air in an inverted U tube connected to a fluid reservoir that drains to a lower elevation. Drainage tends to stop when the continuity of the fluid phase is interrupted by air (Fig. 4–5). Mechanical work per unit weight of fluid (foot pound force per pound of slurry) is equal to z (differential in height from the top of the reservoir to the apex of the U). The patient's intestine apparently was not able to generate this additional force, and the gas lock caused bowel obstruction.

Based on the experience gained in this case we speculate that colonic gas locks are a cause of Ogilvie's syndrome. The hepatic flexure, the splenic flexure, and the sigmoid colon that sustain the greatest directional changes in the colon are the most likely sites for U-tube trapping. This correlates with the most common sites of transition between dilated and nondilated colon (Ogilvie's syndrome).[10] Normal intestinal function and

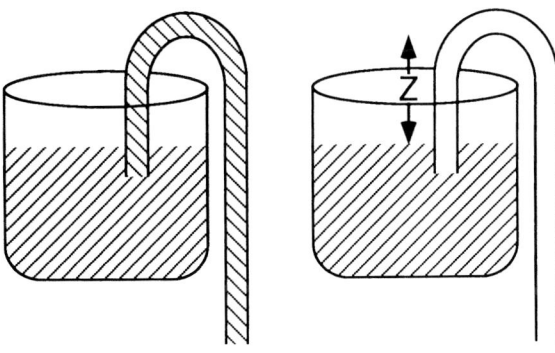

Figure 4–5 Inverted U-tube model showing left free drainage. Right drainage stops when the continuity of the fluid phase is interrupted by air. Mechanical work per unit weight of fluid (foot pound force per pound of slurry) is equal to z (differential in height from the top of the reservoir to the apex of the U).

changes in body position assist in dispersing gas pockets, but when patients are immobilized and/or have impaired intestinal motility—as is the care in the majority of patients with Ogilvie's—colonic gas locks can cause bowel obstruction. Lack of elevated pressure in the gas-locked U opens up the possibility for an attractive yet untested percutaneous approach to management of Ogilvie's. Rather than accessing the cecum, a pressurized site of overflow and back-up, with a tube that drains feces, inserting a small-bore catheter into the atmospherically pressured U loop of colon and aspirating gas could work to restore the natural route of evacuation per rectum. This hypothesis is supported by reports that illustrate successful colonoscopic and transrectal catheter decompression even when the scope cannot be advanced into the dilated segment.[10,24]

CONTRAINDICATIONS

As with most percutaneous procedures, uncorrectable bleeding diathesis is a contraindication for colostomy. Latex allergy may limit the choice of equipment used but not the procedure in general. Similar to percutaneous gastrostomy and jejunostomy, massive ascites and peritoneal dialysis should be considered relative contraindications. The risk of peritoneal spillage is presumed to be increased. Seepage of ascites around the access and retention sutures can cause breakdown of the skin and possibly the enterostomy.[25,26] Patients who cannot assume a supine position can be accessed in a sitting position on the elevated footboard of a radiographic tilt-table.

TECHNICAL CONSIDERATIONS

Puncture of Obstructed vs. Nonobstructed Colon

Accidental puncture of nonobstructed colon during percutaneous nephrostomy occurs uncommonly due to variations in the normal relationship of colon and kidneys, and usually has no long-term sequelae.[27–29] LeRoy et al report two inadvertent colonic transgressions and large-bore dilatation in a series of 1000 percutaneous nephrostomies.[27] An 85-year-old patient with a proximal ureteral stone underwent tract dilatation to 24 Fr for treatment by intracorporeal lithotripsy. A 22-Fr postprocedural nephrostomy tube was left in the renal pelvis. After tube removal, a small amount of feces was noted at the drainage site. CT showed no evidence of abscess or perinephric masses; drainage ceased in 4 days and the patient recovered uneventfully. A similar scenario developed in a 35-year-old woman after placement of a 24-Fr access tract to the left kidney. Intracorporeal lithotripsy was terminated due to a discrepancy between input and output irrigation volumes. Four days later, the patient complained about passing gas through her tube. A CT scan and nephrostogram showed a communication between the nephrostomy tract and the descending colon. A cystoscopic double-J ureteral stent was placed, and the nephrostomy tube was first retracted into the colon and removed several days later. Stool drainage ceased within 24 hours. These cases illustrate that even large tracts placed in a normal and nonobstructed colon are well tolerated without risk of spillage and apparently with rapid tract formation. Such favorable outcome cannot be expected in patients with obstructed colon or altered intestinal wall.

Through the course of performing enterostomies in three patients we conclude that successful and leak-free drainage of distal intestinal obstructions is not straightforward.[20] Subsequently, we developed an in vitro model using porcine gut, which confirmed our clinically gained impressions that (1) an organic obstruction should not be accessed at the site of obstruction; (2) access should be chosen at least 10 cm proximal to the site of obstruction; and (3) the drainage tube should be advanced to the site of obstruction for best decompression and drainage[21] (Fig. 4–6). In our clinical experience, we also found that chronically

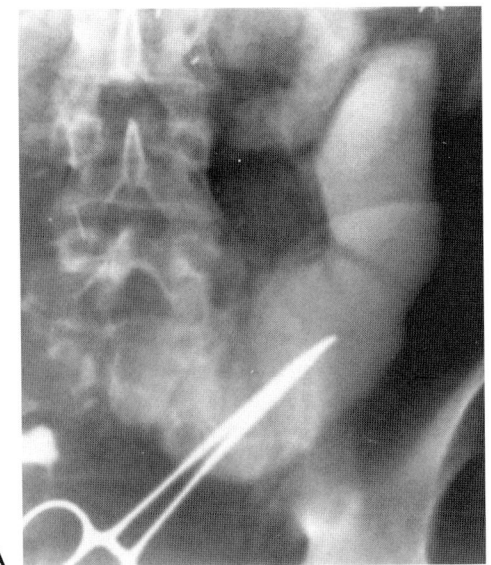
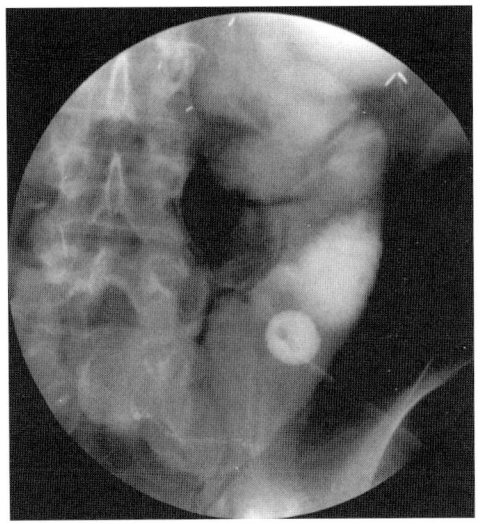

Figure 4–6 A 32-year-old man with amphetamine arteritis and occlusions of the superior mesenteric artery, inferior mesenteric artery, and celiac artery (due to arcuate ligament), and subsequent occlusions of celiac artery and superior mesenteric artery bypass grafts. After colectomy and repeated small bowel resections, only a small segment of bowel was left. The surgical enterostomy scarred down due to ischemia and tube drainage was requested. **(A)** Localization for draining enterostomy. Note distended intestine with distal obstruction. **(B)** Distended intestine at entry site of Foley system and distally. **(C)** Decompression of entry site and distal intestine with distal drainage.

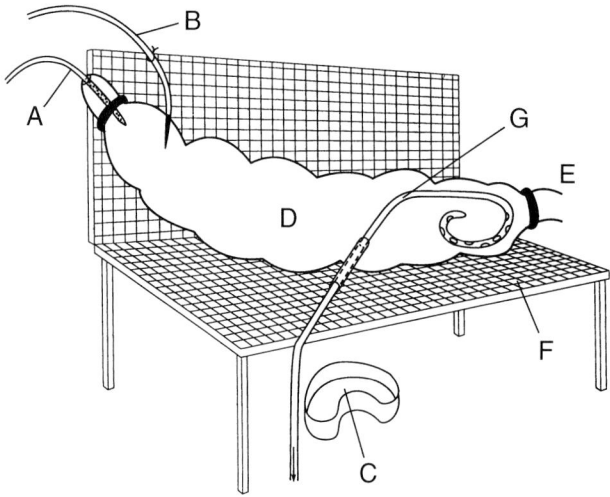

Figure 4–7 Experimental setup. A, inflow tubing; B, spinal needle and pressure tubing; C, leakage receptacle; D, porcine gut; E, distal obstruction site; F, wire stand; G, Thal-Quick drain; H, radially expanding device. (From Carson et al[21], with permission.)

distended and chronically ischemic intestine can be extremely tough in consistency and can pose problems in terms of initial dilatation. On the other hand, previously irradiated intestine can be extremely friable and can disintegrate during access; this resulted in peritonitis and death in one patient.

While entry and tube placement through nonpressurized intestine can probably be considered safe, entry into pressurized colon should only be undertaken after other treatment options have been exhausted.

Maximizing Drainage and Minimizing Leakage

In an effort to evaluate the effects on leakage of access devices, T-tack placement, and location of enterostomy combined with open and closed drainage systems on leakage, we devised an in vitro model using pressurized porcine gut (Fig. 4–7).[21] In this study, initial puncture of pressurized colon and dilatation to 24 Fr with less than 1 mL of spillage was achieved in less than half the trials. Major leakage occurred subsequent to minor technical difficulties, such as wire kinks or slight motion of the dilating assemblies. In this context, stiff or superstiff wires required greater operator experience and were more prone to kinking than medium-stiffness wires.

Pericatheter leakage and intraluminal pressure buildup were unavoidable during closed drainage at the site of obstruction or when the drainage tube was pointed proximally against the stream (Fig. 4–8). Under these conditions, negative pressure tended to suck in the intestinal wall around the ports, resulting in partial or complete obstruction. Only after sufficient intraluminal fluid accumulated and pressure increased were drainage ports freed, and drainage resumed (Fig. 4–9). This may also explain why tubes inserted transrectally past sites of obstruction do not work well. In addition, peristalsis tends to dislodge such tubes.

The sucking in of intestinal wall around the tube ports can be avoided by use of an open-drainage system. In vivo this is only applicable to initial access. Long-term use requires fluid and odor-containing closed systems.

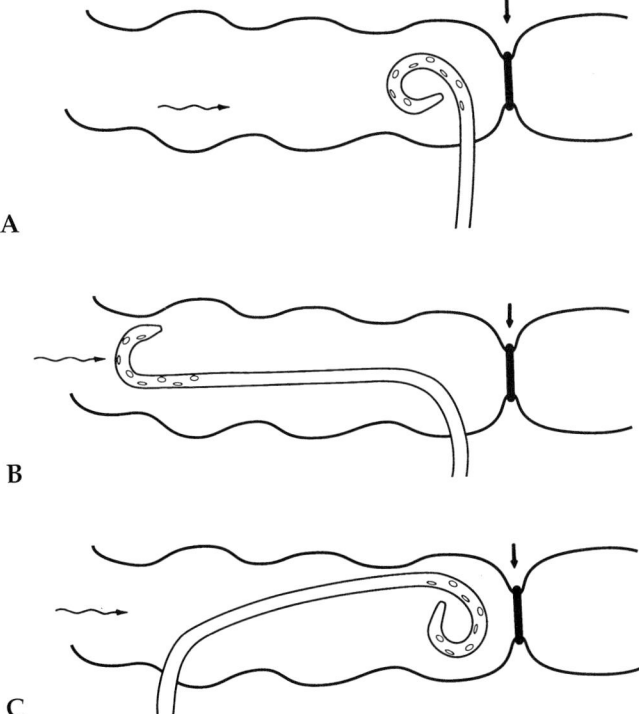

Figure 4–8 Different drainage arrangements. **(A)** Distal access–distal drainage. **(B)** Distal access–proximal drainage. **(C)** Proximal access–distal drainage. *Wavy arrow:* inflow. *Straight arrow:* site of obstruction. (From Carson et al[21], with permission.)

Fixation Devices

A major difficulty with percutaneous enterostomy arises from the lack of fixed apposition between intestine and abdominal wall. Looping of guide wires and catheters in the peritoneal space and leakage of gastric and enteric contents are feared complications of gastrostomy and jejunostomy.[30] These limitations can be overcome by placement of T-tacks or fasteners[30–33] or by observing the indentation of the intestinal wall during entry and forward motions that advance instruments and back motions that bring back the intestinal wall to the abdominal wall (Fig. 4–10). With the latter technique a safe gastrostomy can be achieved without T-tacks.[34] However, the stomach wall is more muscular than that of the remainder of the intestine and therefore is superior in preventing leakage between the tightly opposed drainage tube and muscle layers. During jejunostomy, T-tacks are believed to be essential[33]: they prevent the jejunal loop from moving during catheter placement, obliterate the peritoneal space focally, prevent volvulus of the gut around the catheter, and prevent leakage by allowing adhesions to form following fixation of the jejunum to the anterior abdominal wall. However, one should bear in mind that jejunostomies are usually applied for feeding a nonpressurized system and that T-tacks may not provide the same degree of protection when access into a pressurized system has been attained. T-tacks may decrease the risk of spillage but cannot prevent it altogether, as experience has taught us. T-tacks and retention crossbars have also been associated with an

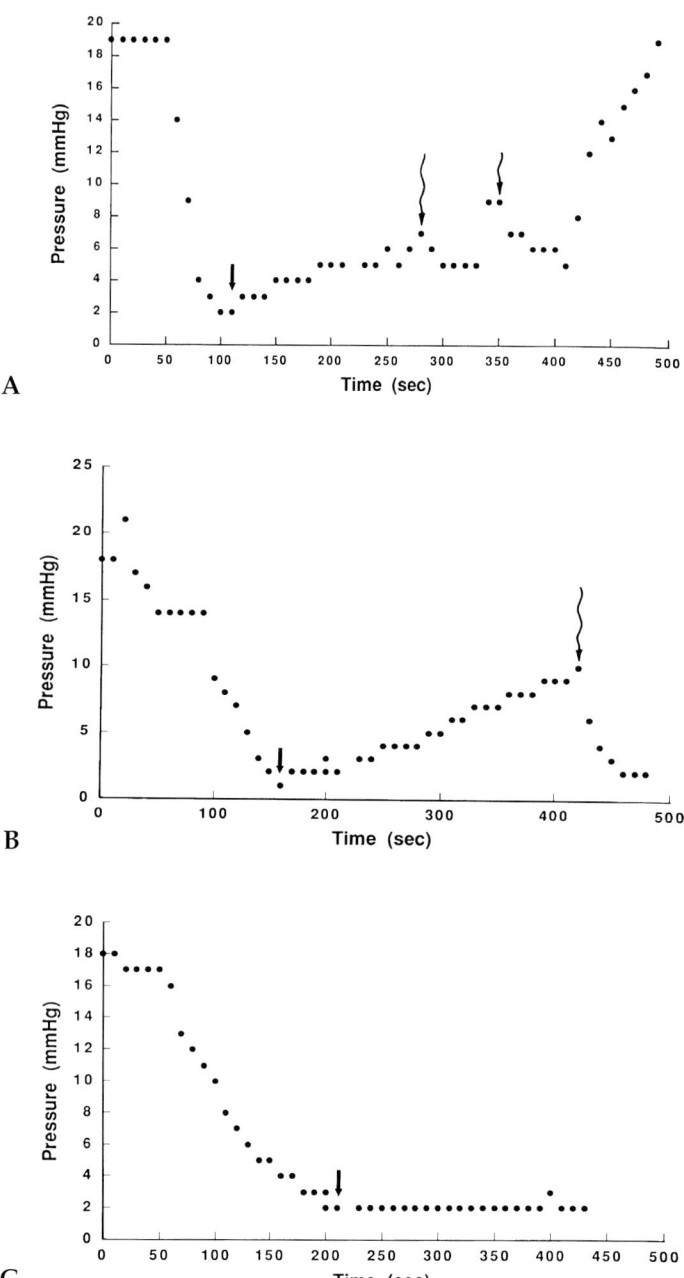

Figure 4–9 Drainage pattern typical of **(A)** distal access–distal drainage and **(B)** distal access–proximal drainage. Straight arrow indicates start of reperfusion at 314 mL/min. Wavy arrow indicates that transient partial drainage resumes only after tube manipulation. **(C)** Drainage pattern typical of proximal access–distal drainage. Arrow indicates start of reperfusion at 314 mL/min. (From Carson et al[21], with permission.)

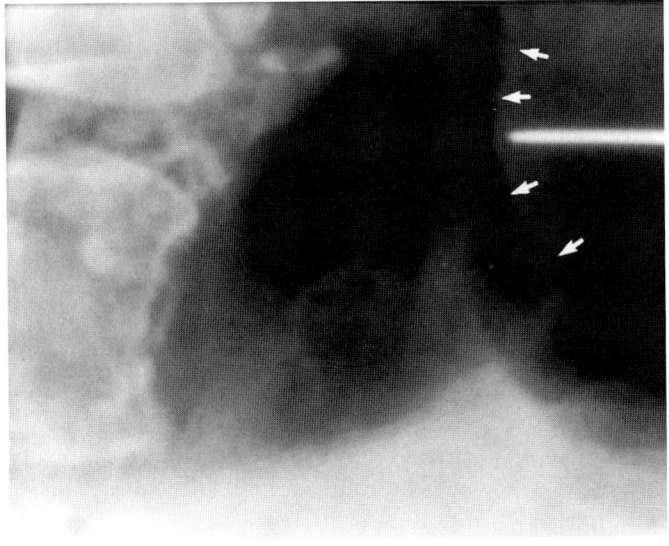

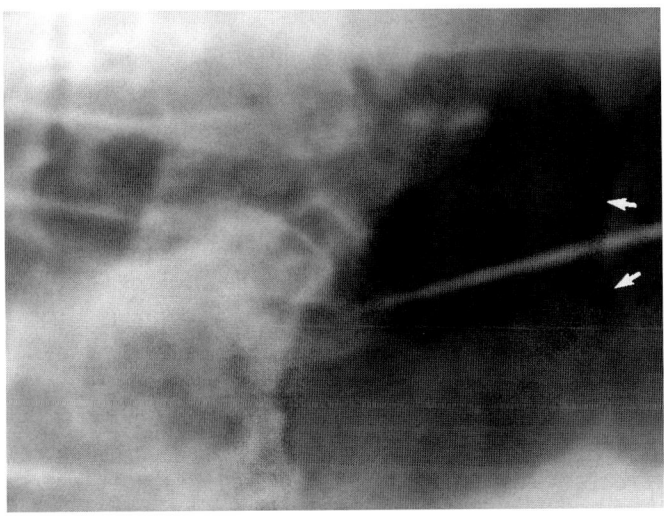

Figure 4–10 Gastric wall (*arrows*) during gastrostomy indentation of stomach wall carried out as part of advancement of puncture needle. **(B)** Retraction of the stomach wall toward the anterior abdominal wall after gentle backward motion of the puncture needle.

increased risk of hemorrhage during fixation of the stomach to the anterior abdominal wall,[35,36] and similar complications may be possible after colonic entry.

T-tacks, employed widely for gastrostomy and jejunostomy, may also be an attractive option for reducing motion and containing leakage during enterostomy. However, our study with isolated pressurized colon showed that T-tacks themselves are associated with a spillage rate of 15 mL/min in pressurized leakage-prone intestine. T-tacks should, therefore, not be anchored in the fluid containing segment of colon if they are used at all during the initial access. Placement in the gas-containing segment is preferable, although decompression of gas through the T-tack entry site may permit the fluid level to raise above the T-tack entry. T-tacks may be helpful after decompression when leakage is no longer a threat and apposition of the intestine to the abdominal wall facilitates tract formation.

Retroperitoneal vs. Transperitoneal Anterior Approach

A retroperitoneal approach theoretically reduces the risk of peritonitis by limiting spillage to the retroperitoneum.[1,14,17] Retroperitoneal spillage can, however, induce severe infectious fasciitis with equally poor or even worse prognosis.[14] The variability in the alignment of the peritoneal reflections makes exact planning of a truly retroperitoneal approach difficult or impossible even under CT guidance.[14,37,38] Poor mobility and massive distention of the colon in the target population further interferes with the interventionalist's ability to access the colon from a retroperitoneal approach, even if such were desired.[14,19] In the supine patient the fluid will accumulate posteriorly and gas will rise anteriorly. A retroperitoneal approach is thus more likely to result in entry into fluid rather than gas. As gas can exit through smaller openings faster than fluid, entry into the gas level permits more rapid decompression while reducing the risk of leakage around the access. The transperitoneal approach is advantageous in debilitated patients who are unable to sustain the prone position. The anterior transperitoneal approach allows anterior fixation of the intestine to the anterior abdominal wall and thus reduces the possibility of fecal leakage. The anterior approach also facilitates tube care. For these reasons, the anterior transabdominal approach is preferable.

Equipment Options

VanSonnenberg et al used fluoroscopy for guidance on four patients with Ogilvie's syndrome and CT on one.[14] They used trocar insertion on two patients and modified Seldinger on three. The catheters used were of various sizes, ranging from 8 to 12 Fr, all with retention devices. Casola et al reporting using CT guidance to introduce a 5-Fr suprapubic cystostomy catheter with a 5-mL balloon using the trocar technique for management of Ogilvie's syndrome.[13] The balloon was inflated immediately after insertion of the catheter, followed by retraction of the catheter to secure the cecum against the anterior abdominal wall. The catheter was then sutured into place after a tight seal was obtained to prevent spillage of fecal materials into the peritoneal space.

Shandling et al report cecostomies in children under intravenous conscious sedation and with glucagon to induce bowel paralysis.[15] The position of the cecum was localized under fluoroscopy. A 19-gauge, 7-cm single-wall puncture needle loaded with a gastric retention suture was introduced and deployed using a 0.025-in. guide wire. The cecum was secured to the anterior abdominal wall. A 4-Fr sheath and dilator was introduced, followed by a second retention suture, which also secured the cecum to the anterior abdominal wall. A 10-Fr fascial dilator was introduced to dilate the tract and a 10-Fr cope catheter with a retention loop was introduced. The catheter was then retracted to oppose the cecum to the anterior abdominal wall. The procedure was further modified with a trap-door device at the puncture site to minimize tube bulk and provide easy access.

Patel et al used a 16-gauge intracatheter needle to access and decompress a cecal volvulus with an anterior approach, following localization of the dilated cecum with plain abdominal radiographs and a cross-table lateral.[18] The catheter was withdrawn within minutes after immediate cecal deflation.

Morrison et al report the percutaneous placement of a 24-Fr Foley catheter into the cecum using Seldinger's technique.

There are very few reports in the literature describing the use of percutaneous colostomies for the drainage of stool. However, Morrison et al reportedly drained 5 L of liquid stool over 72 hours. Nonemergency surgery followed one week later for probable iatrogenic obstruction of the transverse colon following cholecystectomy with partial resection of the duodenum and transverse colon.[19]

SUGGESTED APPROACH

As pointed out above, most experience with percutaneous colostomy has been anecdotal, with the exception of a large series pertaining to fecal irrigation. Recommendations are therefore based on both reported experience and conceptual deductions thereof. The following recommendations are to be seen only as guidelines in this evolving field of intervention.

First a distinction should be made as to whether the colon is pressurized. Interventional technique is chosen accordingly. General considerations apply to any colostomy.

General Considerations

Patient sedation may not be required as long as local anesthesia is applied. Given patient-to-patient variability with respect to pain and anxiety, short-acting parenteral analgesic may be required. Since patients undergoing colostomy are, by the nature of their referral, often in a critical clinical condition, nonpharmacologic adjuncts in the form of self-hypnotic relaxation and imagery may be helpful in reducing or eliminating intravenous sedatives and narcotics.[39] Patients with distended intestine are at risk from aspiration; therefore, provisions for suctioning and/or functioning nasogastric tubes should be in place. When massive distention produces marked diaphragmatic elevation and impairs breathing in the supine position, patients can be treated while sitting on the elevated footboard of an upright fluoroscopy tilt-table. Because of the risk of fecal spillage, intravenous antibiotic prophylaxis is recommended.

Whether CT or fluoroscopy is used, a direct anterior approach to an air-containing segment of intestine is recommended. During choice of the entry site attention should be paid to the location of the inferior epigastric artery to avoid its puncture and bleeding during the initial puncture and dilation. A skin incision large enough to accept the chosen access devices is made and a subcutaneous tract created with blunt hemostat dissection without violation of the peritoneum or the adjacent intestine. Puncture with a Seldinger needle or trocar should be brief and deliberate once the access site has been determined, reducing tenting of the colonic wall. The position of the needle should be confirmed by aspiration of air or fecal contents combined with repeat axial images at that level or biplane fluoroscopy. A Rosen or Bentson guide wire is then introduced through the needle and directed to the site of obstruction. If devices with retention balloons are used, the balloon can be inflated immediately after insertion and retracted backward to provide a tight seal between the colon and the abdominal wall. Depending on the purpose of the procedure (irrigation versus drainage), larger bore tubes can be used (e.g., 24- to 30-Fr Quick Thal (Cook, Inc., Bloomington, IN) drainage tubes).

Organic Bowel Obstruction

In the presence of an organic bowel obstruction, the following recommendations are made:

1. Access should be at least 10 cm proximal to the site of obstruction (Fig. 4-8).
2. Initial dilatation can best be done with a one-step dilatation device that can be inserted with little motion and possesses an inner sealant balloon. Complete familiarity with the device

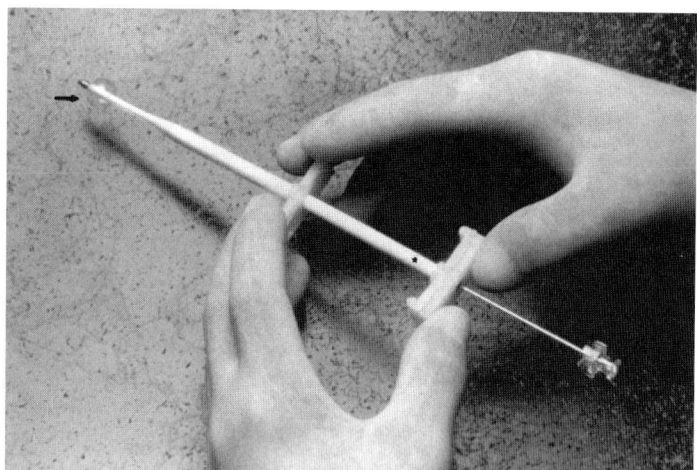

Figure 4–11 Radially expanding dilator. Arrow points to inflatable balloon at the tip. Dilatation is accomplished via coaxial advancement of an inner dilator (*) through an outer sheath combination. (From Carson et al[21], with permission.)

and preprocedure practice are essential. Unfortunately, the only commercially available one-step device that dilates to 24 Fr (R.E.D. InnerDyne, Mountain View, CA) has been altered by the manufacturer for use during laparoscopic procedures and hence is no longer useful for colostomy (Fig. 4–11). A less desirable but available alternative for large-bore dilatation is to use a 24-Fr Amplatz dilator coaxially loaded over an 8-mm balloon (Fig. 4–12).

3. Initial drainage should be open until the colon is entirely decompressed.
4. A large-bore tube with additional sideholes is advanced toward the site of obstruction to decompress the puncture site.
5. T-tacks that secure the tract are applied after the intestine has been entirely decompressed.

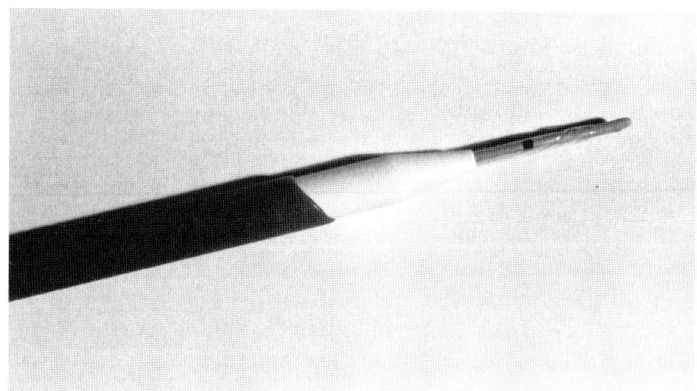

Figure 4–12 Combination of an 8-mm angioplasty balloon and an Amplatz sheath. (From Carson et al[21], with permission.)

Nonobstructed, Nondilated Colon

Smaller bore access devices can be used. If the intestine is not distended it may not abut the abdominal wall. Intravenous glucagon is useful for paralysis of the intestine and may also bring the colon closer to the entry site. CT guidance may be advisable if the anatomical relationships at the chosen entry site cannot be fully defined under fluoroscopy. T-tacks may be needed early on to provide sufficient stability during tract dilatation.

Ogilvie's Syndrome

Technique depends on whether Ogilvie's syndrome presents predominantly as a massively dilated air-filled cecum or as an obstruction with air-fluid levels. Cecal decompression in the former instance may be all that is needed, provided the rapid intestinal pressure change also abolishes any operational gas locks. If drainage is required in the presence of extensive air-fluid levels, an approach as in bowel obstruction may be safer. However, the most attractive alternative would be to access the gas lock in the inverted U with a small-bore tube, thus restoring the patient's ability to evacuate per rectum.

Postprocedure Management

Serial abdominal films and close monitoring of the patient's vital signs should be obtained for early detection of peritonitis or recurrent colonic distention. Dressing changes should be made daily, with close observations for skin breakdown and leakage at the access site. Depending on the underlying pathophysiology, it may be necessary to aspirate gas actively. Minimal bulking meals or feedings should be given to prevent occlusion of draining enterostomies. If tubes remain solely for irrigation or aspiration of air, dietary intake need be adjusted only if accompanying diseases require it.

Summary

Percutaneous colostomy is a relatively noninvasive alternative to surgical colostomy that has been used in the management of distal bowel obstruction. Clinical applications have included cecal decompression in Ogilvie's syndrome, colonic irrigation for management of fecal incontinence and for delivery of antibiotics, detorsion of cecal volvulus, and management of intestinal gas lock. Most experience with percutaneous colostomy has been anecdotal. Consequently, indications and techniques for its use are still evolving. With further understanding, experience, and availability of appropriate access devices, increased use of the procedure can be anticipated. With the given suggestions in mind, a relatively safe approach to colostomy should be feasible.

References

1. Crass JR, Simmons RL, Frick MP, Maile CW. Percutaneous decompression of the colon using CT guidance in Ogilvie syndrome. *Am J Roentgenol* 1985;144:475–476.
2. Nanni C, Garbini A, Luchetti P, Nanni G, Ronconi P, Castagneto M. Ogilvie syndrome (acute colonic pseudo-obstruction). *Dis Colon Rectum* 1982;25:157–165.
3. Vanek VW, Al-Salti M. Acute pseudo obstruction of the colon (Ogilvie's syndrome): an analysis of 400 cases. *Dis Colon Rectum* 1986;29:203–210.
4. Johnson CD, Rice RP, Kelvin FM, Foster WL, Williford ME. The radiologic evaluation of gross cecal distension. *Am J Roentgenol* 1985;145:1211–1217.
5. Rahbar A, Easley GW, Mendoza CB Jr. Volvulus of the cecum. *Am Surg* 1973;39:325–330
6. Grover NK, Gulati SM, Tagor NK. Volvulus of the cecum and ascending colon. *Am J Surg* 1973;125:672–675.
7. Ogilvie H. Large-intestine colic due to sympathetic deprivation: a new clinical syndrome. *Br J Med* 1948;2:671–673.
8. Dunlop JA. Ogilvie's syndrome or false colonic obstruction. *Br Med J* 1949;5:890–891.

9. Strodel WE, Nostrant TT, Eckhauser FE, Dent TL. Therapeutic and diagnostic colonoscopy in nonobstructive colonic dilatation. *Ann Surg* 1983;197:416–421.
10. Bode WE, Beart RW, Spencer RJ, Culp CE, Wolff BG, Taylor BM. Colonoscopic decompression for acute pseudo obstruction of the colon: report of 22 cases and review of the literature. *Am J Surg* 1984;147:243–245.
11. VanZwalenburd CV. Strangulation resulting from distension of hollow viscera. *Ann Surg* 1907;46:780–786.
12. Nivatvongs S, Vermeulen FD, Fang DT. Colonoscopic decompression of acute pseudo-obstruction of the colon. *Ann Surg* 1982;196:598–600.
13. Casola G, Withers C, vanSonnenberg E, Herba MJ, Saba RM, Brown RA. Percutaneous cecostomy for decompression of the massively distended cecum. *Radiology* 1986; 158:793–794.
14. VanSonnenberg E, Varney RR, Casola G, et al. Percutaneous cecostomy for Ogilvie syndrome: laboratory observations and clinical experience. *Radiology* 1990;175:679–682.
15. Shandling B, Chait PG, Richards HF. Percutaneous cecostomy: a technique in the management of fecal incontinence. *J Pediatr Surg* 1996;31:534–537.
16. Chait PG, Shandling B, Richards HM, Connolly BL. Fecal incontinence in children: treatment with percutaneous cecostomy tube: a prospective study. *Radiology* 1997; 203:621–624.
17. Haaga JR, Bick RJ, Zollinger RM. CT guided percutaneous catheter cecostomy. *Gastrointest Radiol* 1987;12:166–168.
18. Patel D, Berman MD, Ansari E. Percutaneous decompression of cecal volvulus. *Am J Roentgenol* 1987;148:747–748
19. Morrison MC, Stafford SA, Saini S, Mueller PR. Percutaneous cecostomy: controlled transperitoneal approach. *Radiology* 1990; 176:574–576.
20. Lang EV. Technical consideration for percutaneous placement of distal draining enterostomies. *Radiology* 1994;193(P):134.
21. Carson L, Lang EV. Percutaneous colostomy for treatment of mechanical bowel obstruction. *J Vasc Interv Radiol* 1996;7: 561–567.
22. Mainar A, Tejero E, Maynar M, Ferral H, Castaneda-Zuniga W. Colorectal obstruction: treatment with metallic stents. *Radiology* 1996;198:761–764.
23. Canon CL, Baron TH, Morgan DE, Dean PA, Koehler RE. Treatment of colonic obstruction with metallic stents: radiologic features. *Am J Roentgenol* 1997;168:199–205.
24. Bender GN, Do-Dai DD, Briggs LM. Colonic pseudo-obstruction: decompression with a tricomponent coaxial system under fluoroscopic guidance. *Radiology* 1993;188:395–398.
25. Lee MJ, Saini S, Brink JA, Morrison MC, Hahn PF, Mueller PR. Malignant small bowel obstruction and ascites: not a contraindication to percutaneous gastrostomy. *Clin Radiol* 1991;44:332–334.
26. McFarland EG, Lee MJ, Boland GW, Mueller PR. Gastropexy breakdown and peritonitis after percutaneous gastrojejunostomy in a patient with ascites. *Am J Roentgenol* 1994; 164:189–193.
27. LeRoy AJ, Williams HH, Bender CE, Segura JW, Paterson DE, Benson RC. Colon perforation following nephrostomy and renal calculus removal. *Radiology* 1985;155:83–85.
28. Almgard LE, Fernström I. Percutaneous nephropyelostomy. *Acta Radiol* 1974;15:288–293.
29. Hildell J, Aspelin P, Sigfússon B. Percutaneous nephrostomy: aspects on clinical application. *Acta Radiol (Diagn)* 1980;21:485–490.
30. Brown AS, Mueller PR, Ferrucci JTJ. Controlled percutaneous gastrostomy: nylon T-fasteners for fixation of the anterior gastric wall. *Radiology* 1986;158:543–545.
31. Shellito PC, Malt RA. Tube gastrostomy: technique and complications. *Ann Surg* 1985; 201:180–195.
32. Saini S, Mueller PR, Gaa J, et al. Percutaneous gastrostomy with gastropexy: experience in 125 patients. *Am J Roentgenol* 1990;154:1003–1006.
33. Gray R, Rooney M, Grosman H. Use of T-fasteners for primary jejunostomy. *Cardiovasc Intervent Radiol* 1990;13:93–94.
34. Hicks ME, Surratt RS, Marx MV, Picus D, Lang EV. Fluoroscopically guided percutaneous gastrostomy and gastroenterostomy: analysis of 158 consecutive cases. *Am J Roentgenol* 1990;154:725–728.
35. DiSario JA, Foutch PG, Sanowski RA. Poor results with percutaneous endoscopic jejunostomy. *Gastrointest Endosc* 1990;36: 257–260.

36. Deutsch LS, Kannegieter L, Vanson D, Miller D, Brandon J. Simplified percutaneous gastrostomy. *Radiology* 1992;184:181–183.
37. Rubenstein WA, Auh YH, Zirinsky K, Kneeland JB, Whalen JP, Kazam E. Posterior peritoneal recesses: assessment using CT. *Radiology* 1995;156:461–468.
38. Quinn SF, Jones EN, Maroney T. Percutaneous cecostomy in the management of cecal volvulus—report of a case. *J Vasc Interv Radiol* 1987;2:137–139.
39. Lang EV, Joyce JS, Spiegel D, Hamilton D, Lee K. Self-hypnotic relaxation during interventional radiological procedures: effects on pain perception and intravenous drug use. *Int J Exp Clin Hyp* 1996;44:106–119.

Chapter 5

Peritoneal/Retroperitoneal Anatomy: Relevance to Performance of Interventional Procedures

John P. McGahan
R. Brooke Jeffrey, Jr.
Michael J. Lane

INTRODUCTION

Understanding the compartmental anatomy of the abdomen is of profound importance to the proper performance of percutaneous interventional procedures. It is necessary to understand the peritoneal and retroperitoneal anatomy of the abdomen to prepare for guidance of interventional therapy and to avoid potential pitfalls. For instance, when performing aspiration or drainage of pelvic fluid collection, it is necessary to know compartmental anatomy to understand the possible origins of fluid collections. A pelvic fluid collection may be secondary to a number of conditions including such primary pelvic diseases as a tubo-ovarian abscess; however, the pelvic fluid collection may have spread to the pelvis from another site. As there is free communication from both the right and left pericolic gutter to the pelvic cul-de-sac, the fluid collection may be secondary to an appendiceal or diverticular abscess (Fig. 5–1). Drainage of the pelvic abscess is unlikely to be curative if the primary abnormality, the appendiceal or diverticular abscess, is overlooked.

As another example, placement of abscess drainage catheters from one abdominal or retroperitoneal compartment to another should be avoided at certain times. Often the most direct route for drainage of a subdiaphragmatic abscess may be through the pleura into the subdiaphragmatic space. However, this route should be avoided to prevent the spread of infection to the pleural cavity. Knowledge of the anatomical relationship of the pleural space to the subdiaphragmatic space is needed to avoid this pitfall.

This chapter will review the compartmental anatomy of the abdomen and pelvis needed to best perform percutaneous interventional procedures. The chapter will also cover paths of fluid spread and compartmental localization of abdominal abscesses. Potential pitfalls to avoid in performing percutaneous drainage of abdominal pelvic fluid collections will be presented. Complete knowledge of abdominal compartmental anatomy should be obtained by any clinician planning to perform percutaneous interventional procedures.

SUPRADIAPHRAGMATIC VS. SUBDIAPHRAGMATIC FLUID COLLECTION

Although it may seem elementary to determine if fluid is in the pleural cavity or the abdomen, at times this distinction is

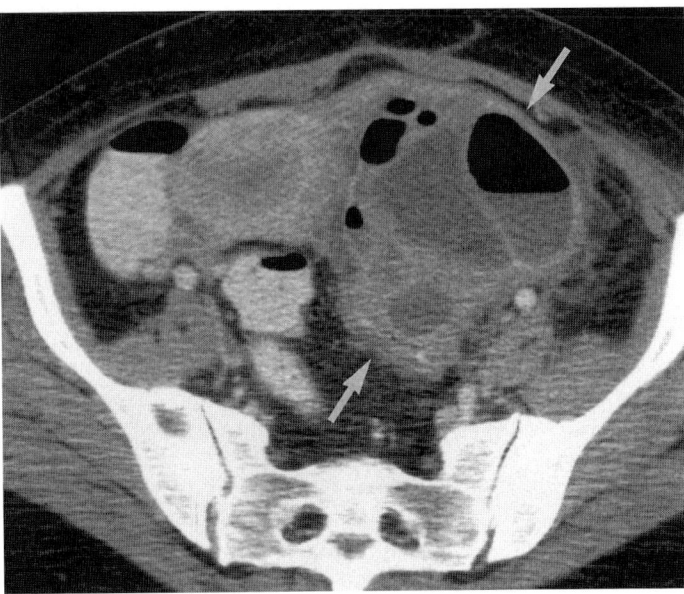

Figure 5–1 Diverticular abscess mimicking a tubo-ovarian abscess (TOA). Contrast-enhanced computed tomogram in a 44-year-old woman with left lower quadrant (LLQ) pain, fever, and a history of pelvic inflammatory disease shows a complex fluid collection in the LLQ with numerous gas-liquid levels (*arrows*). The initial impression was that this mass represented a TOA. Diverticulitis was considered in the differential diagnosis. The lesion was drained and the patient improved. A subsequent barium enema showed numerous diverticula and communication with the abscess cavity. Sigmoid diverticulitis was confirmed surgically.

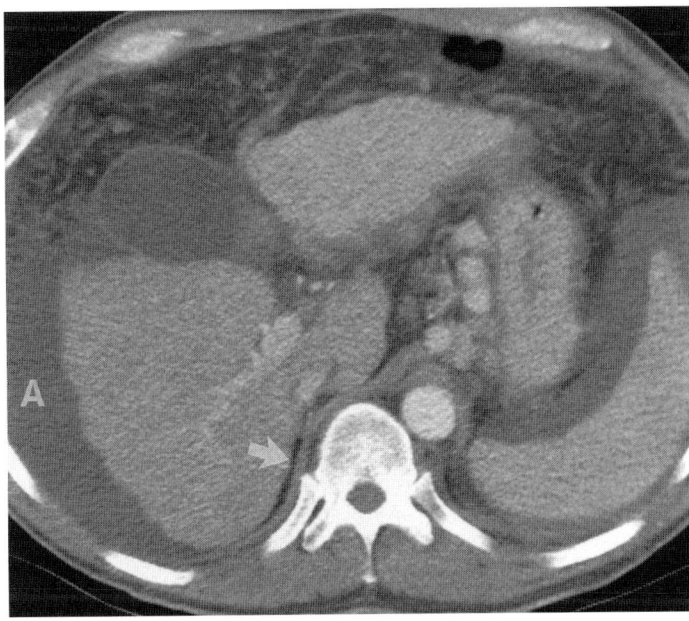

Figure 5–2 Bare area of the liver. Contrast-enhanced computed tomogram in a 65-year-old man with cirrhosis, ascites (A), and varices shows the thin layer of fat (*arrow*) between the bare area of the liver and the diaphragm.

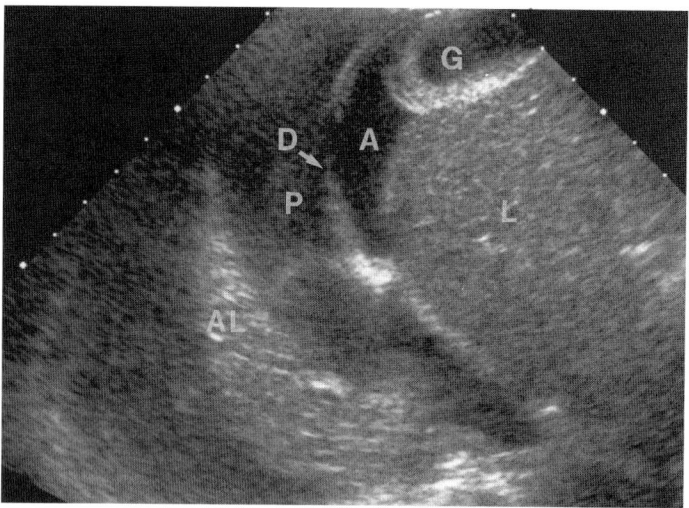

Figure 5–3 Parasagittal sonography of the right upper quadrant (RUQ) clarifies anatomical relationships of fluid collections. Longitudinal sonogram of the RUQ in a 61-year-old man with cirrhosis shows three separate fluid collections, including the gallbladder (G), intraperitoneal ascites (A), and a large pleural effusion (P) adjacent to atelectatic lung (AL), diaphragm (D), and liver (L).

difficult. Knowledge of fluid location is important when performing any drainage procedure to determine the specific path for needle or catheter placement. Four values (1–4) are used to describe the location of fluid relative to the diaphragm.[1–4] These values are assigned as follows:

1. *"Bare area" sign.* There is a bare area of the liver bounded by the coronary ligaments in which the liver is directly attached to the diaphragm and the posterior abdominal wall. Intraperitoneal fluid cannot accumulate posterior to the liver, and any fluid observed in this area on imaging lies within the pleural space (Fig. 5–2).
2. *"Interface" sign.* The interface between peritoneal fluid and the liver is sharp and well defined, whereas the interface between pleural fluid and liver is poorly defined. Unsharpness is probably secondary to the thickness of the diaphragm and volume averaging of curved surfaces that is influenced by slice thickness.
3. *"Displaced crus" sign.* If the medial aspect of the diaphragmatic crura is displaced away from the spine, fluid collection is pleural in position. Fluid that lies lateral and anterior to the diaphragmatic crus is intraperitoneal in position.
4. *"Diaphragm" sign.* On an axial CT scan, fluid that lies below or inside the diaphragm is subdiaphragmatic in location, whereas fluid that lies posterior or outside the diaphragm is pleural in position.

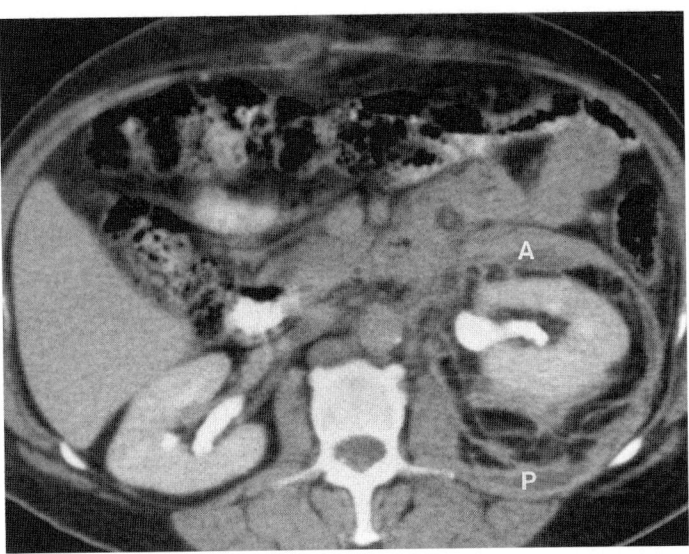

Figure 5–4 Perinephric septa. Contrast-enhanced computed tomogram of a 65-year-old man with pancreatitis shows communication between the anterior (A) and posterior (P) interfacial compartments as well as fluid and/or digestive enzymes from the pancreas. It remains unclear whether the septa act as a barrier or as a conduit in communication between the perinephric space and the interfacial planes anteriorly and posteriorly.

Parasagittal ultrasound is helpful in showing the relationship of the fluid to the diaphragm (Fig. 5–3).

RETROPERITONEUM

Fluid collections or abscesses may be located in the retroperitoneum. Understanding the anatomy of the retroperitoneum and those structures that border potential spaces is important in determining the location of abnormal fluid collections. Understanding of the compartmental anatomy of the abdomen is important to ensure complete treatment. As an example, pancreatic pseudocysts may dissect into different peritoneal and retroperitoneal compartments (Figs. 5–4 and 5–5). Percutaneous drainage of the infected pancreatic pseudocysts may not be curative unless the multiple localized collections in various peritoneal or retroperitoneal compartments are adequately

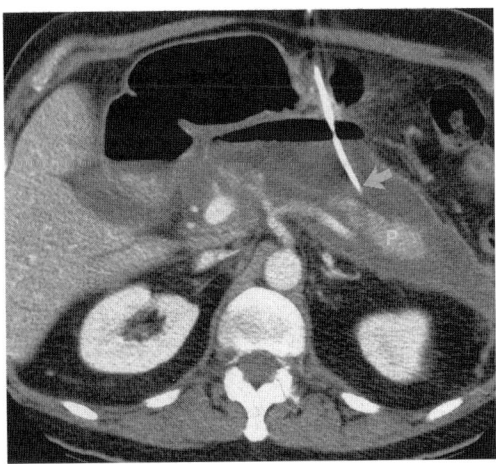

Figure 5–5 Necrotic pancreatic abscess. Contrast-enhanced computed tomogram in 63-year-old man who presented with sepsis shows a drainage catheter (*arrow*) inserted in an anterior pararenal space abscess. A large gas-liquid level is seen in the anterior pararenal space along with a small amount of enhancing pancreatic tissue (P).

CHAPTER 5 • PERITONEAL/RETROPERITONEAL ANATOMY

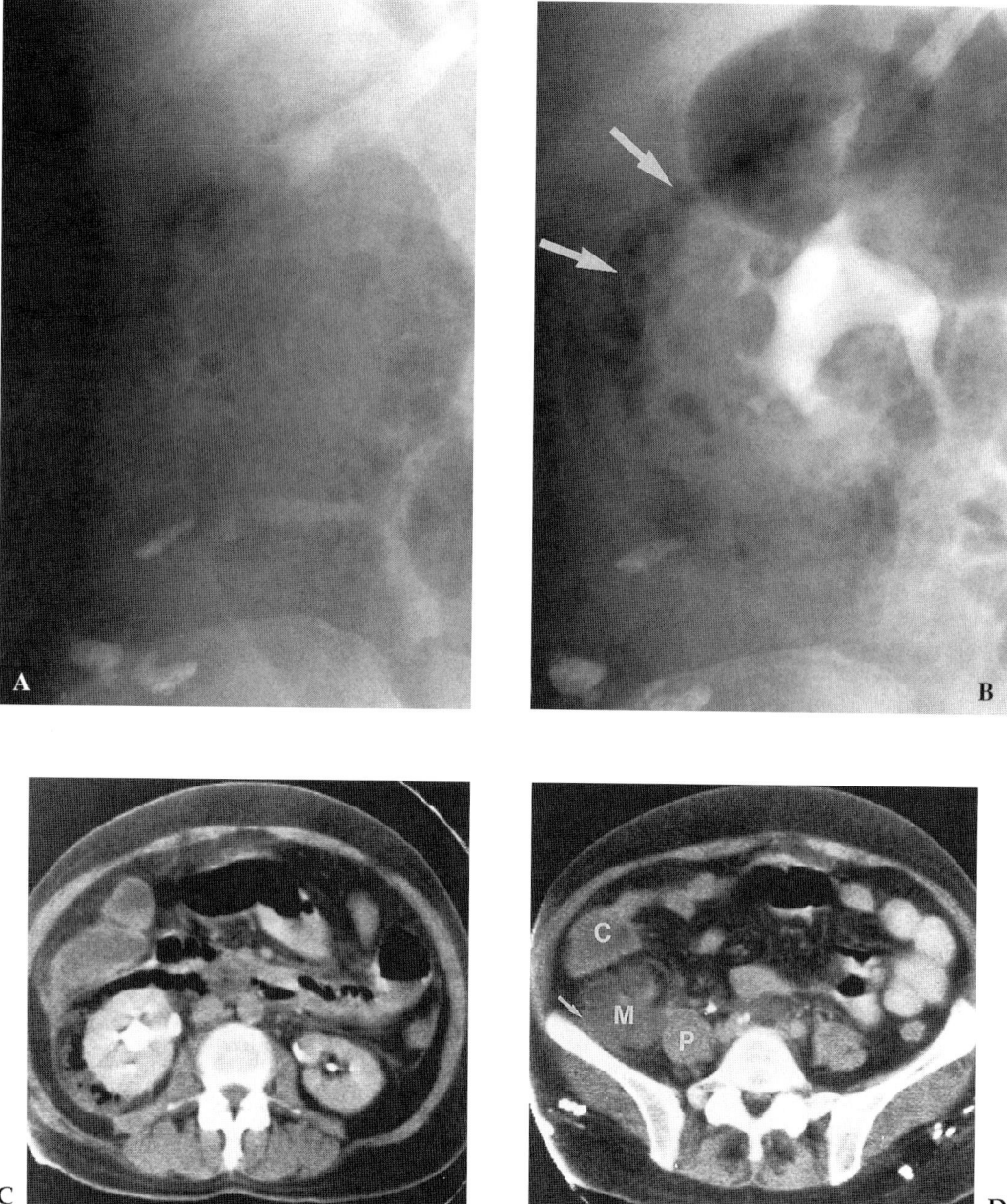

Figure 5–6 Perinephric abscess secondary to ruptured retrocecal appendix. **(A)** Plain film showing stippled collection of gas overlying right kidney. **(B)** Excretory urogram demonstrating stippled gas in perinephric space with distention of fat containing perinephric space (*arrows*). **(C)** Gas and fluid in right perinephric space. **(D)** Mass (M) inferior to right kidney and posterior to ascending colon (C) corresponding to an appendiceal abscess, which causes obliteration of iliacus and psoas (P) muscle. This demonstrates potential communication between the retroperitoneal spaces. Treatment of the obvious perinephric collection would have not been curative, and drainage of appendiceal abscess was necessary. (From McGahan JP. Perinephric abscess secondary to ruptured retrocecal appendix diagnosed by computerized tomography. *Urology* 1982;19: 217–219, with permission).

drained. Without effective drainage of all compartments, percutaneous therapy will probably fail.

Figure 5–6 is an example of multicompartmental involvement by an abscess. The patient presented with what was initially thought to be primary perinephric abscess. However, CT scanning showed the primary abnormality to be a periappendiceal abscess from a ruptured retrocecal appendix. This then ruptured into the perinephric space.

Anatomy

The retroperitoneum is divided by renal fascia into three distinct compartments.[2,5,6] These include (1) the perirenal space, (2) the anterior pararenal space, and (3) the posterior pararenal space.

Perirenal Space

The perirenal or perinephric space is bordered anteriorly by the anterior renal (Gerota's) fascia and posteriorly by the posterior renal (Zuckerkandel's) fascia (Fig. 5–7). The posterior layer of the posterior renal fascia continues anterolaterally to form the lateroconal fascia. Medially, the anterior renal fascia blends with the connective tissues surrounding the great vessels. Usually there is no communication across the midline between the two perirenal spaces. The perirenal space contains the kidney, the adrenal

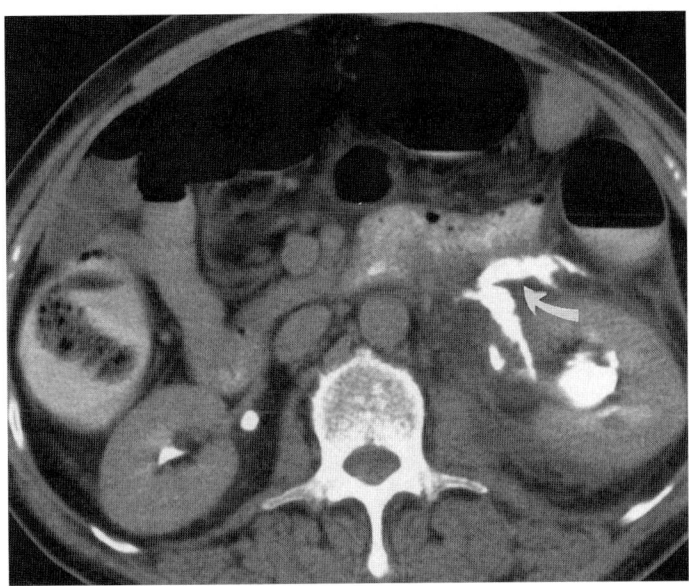

Figure 5–7 Contrast extravasation into the perinephric space. Contrast-enhanced computed tomogram in a 69-year-old man with a history of sigmoid diverticulitis resulting in distal left ureteral obstruction and hydronephrosis who now presents with increasing left flank pain. Shown is extravasation of intravenous contrast material into the perinephric space (*arrow*) from a presumed ruptured fornix. Note how the contrast material is bounded anteriorly by the anterior interfascial space.

gland, the renal vessels, the proximal ureter, and variable amounts of fat. There is a network of bridging septae that extend between the renal capsule and the renal fascia. The septae potentially limit the spread of pathologic processes in the perirenal space.

Anterior Pararenal Space

The anterior pararenal space is bordered by the posterior parietal peritoneum, posteriorly by the anterior renal fascia, and laterally by the lateroconal fascia. The anterior pararenal space contains the pancreas, the duodenum, and the ascending and descending colon (Fig. 5–8). Infection from any of these organs may spread into the retroperitoneal spaces.

Understanding retroperitoneal anatomy is important when performing interventional procedures for several reasons. Knowledge of which organs lie in the anterior pararenal space is important to better localize the potential source of abnormality. Also, as the point of fusion of the anterior and posterior renal fascia is variable, the ascending or descending colon extends posterior to the kidney in approximately 2% of subjects in the supine position and up to 10% of subjects in the prone position. Awareness of this fact is very important, especially when performing

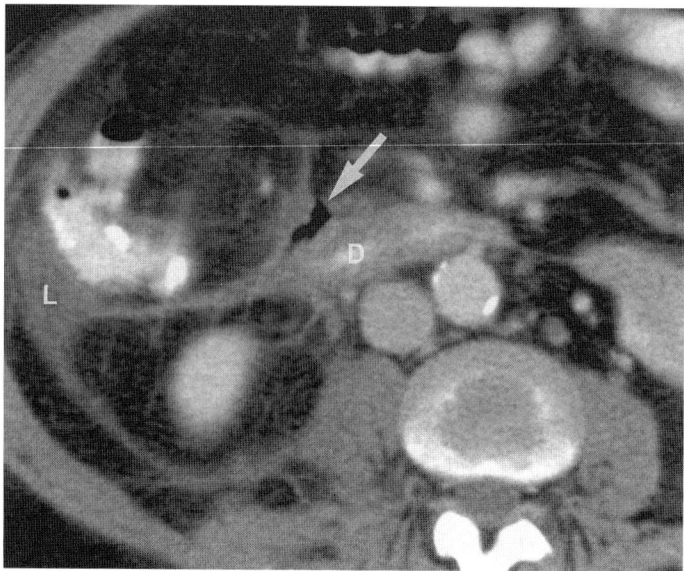

Figure 5–8 Retroperitoneal perforation of the duodenum. Contrast-enhanced computed tomogram in a 63-year-old with abdominal pain following endoscopic retrograde cholangiopancreatography shows a small amount of free gas (*arrow*) adjacent to the duodenal (D) sweep, indicating a perforation. Also shown is bowel content tracking into the anterior and posterior interfascial planes, which are communicating with the lateroconal fascia (L). This emphasizes the retroperitoneal position of the proximal duodenum and its position in the anterior pararenal space.

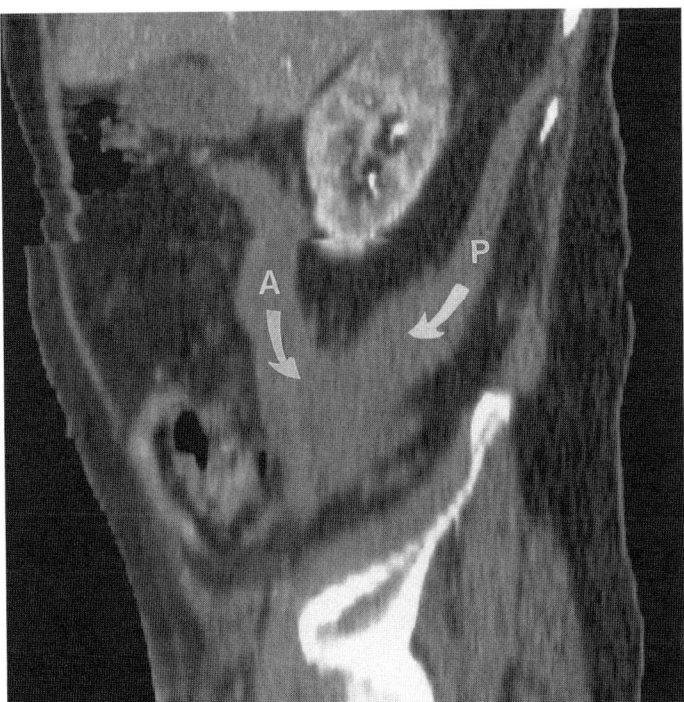

Figure 5–9 Aortic rupture. Result of contrast-enhanced computed tomography with sagittal reformation in a 71-year-old man shows the fat in the perinephric space outlined by blood in the anterior (A) and posterior (B) interfascial compartments of the retroperitoneum. These compartments extend inferiorly (*arrows*) as a cone as they track toward the pelvis.

procedures such as percutaneous nephrostomy. If the retrorenal colon is not observed prospectively, then the catheter may inadvertently traverse the colon.[7,8]

Posterior Pararenal Space
The posterior renal space is bordered anteriorly and medially by the posterior renal and the lateroconal fascia. It is bounded posteriorly and laterally by the transversalis fascia. The posterior pararenal space continues anteriorly as the properitoneal fat line, which is identified as a lucent band on plain abdominal radiographs. Inferiorly, in the pelvis, the anterior and posterior renal fascia are usually incompletely fused and thus may allow extension of fluid from these spaces to the pelvis (Fig. 5–9). Understanding of these different compartmental anatomies is important because fluid and/or abscess can extend from one to another retroperitoneal space. For instance, fluid and debris from pancreatic necrosis may extend from the anterior pararenal space to the posterior pararenal space[5] (Fig. 5–4). This anatomical relationship is important because satisfactory percutaneous drainage requires drainage of the fluid collected in each pararenal space.

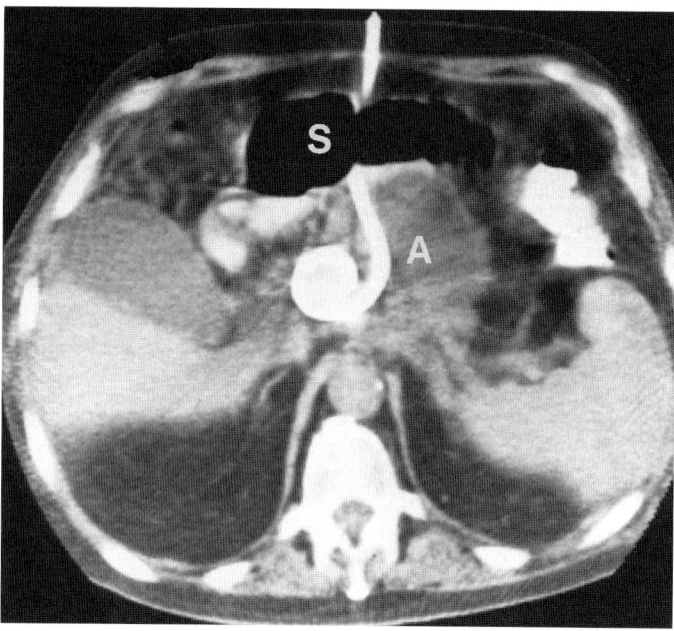

Figure 5–10 Well-demarcated pancreatic abscess (A) located in the lesser sac. Route chosen for drainage is the transgastric route with the catheter placed percutaneously through the stomach (S) and into the pancreatic abscess (A). Computed tomography was used to avoid catheter transgression of the transverse colon.

PERITONEUM

Understanding the peritoneal anatomy is critical to the performance of percutaneous interventional procedures. As a simple example, the lesser sac is bounded by both the stomach and the transverse colon. Although transgression of the stomach for either diagnostic or therapeutic drainage is an accepted approach, in no instance should the colon be violated during percutaneous drainage because it has a high bacterial count (Fig. 5–10). The anatomical relationships must be known prior to performance of percutaneous interventional procedures.

Also, understanding pathways of communication within anatomical compartments is a prerequisite to diagnosing the potential source of infection and its extent. For instance, massive intra-abdominal free fluid, hemorrhage, or abscess formation can spread to the pelvis through normal anatomical pathways. When performing imaging procedures prior to percutaneous therapy, visualization of the pelvis is often required to determine the full extent of abdominal fluid collections and plan the most effective therapy.

Anatomy

The abdominal peritoneal cavity refers to the abdomen proper, consisting of the greater peritoneal cavity (greater sac) and the lesser peritoneal cavity (lesser sac)[6,9,10] (Fig. 5–11). The upper peritoneal cavity communicates freely with the pelvis. The pelvic cul-de-sac is the most dependent

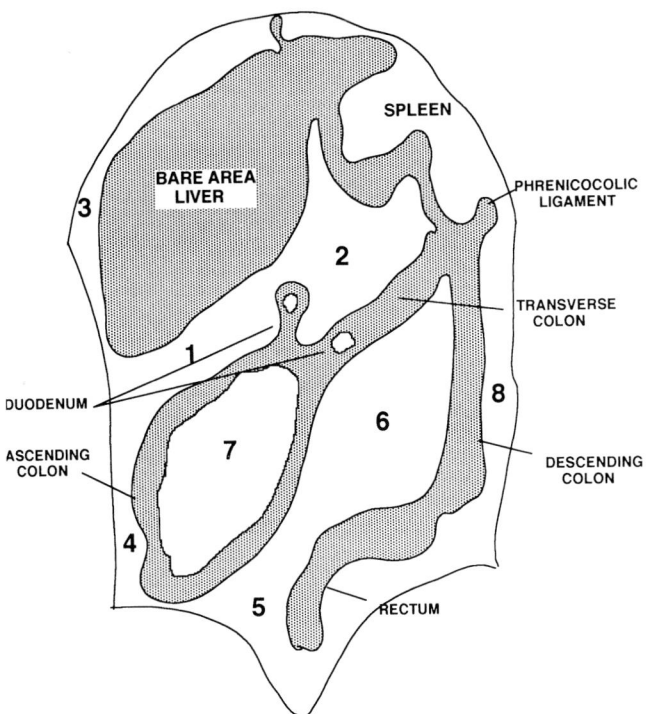

Figure 5–11 Spread of fluid between the different intraperitoneal compartments. For instance, fluid in the hepatorenal fossa, Morrison's pouch (1), may spread to the lesser sac (2) through the foramen of Winslow. Fluid also may spread from the hepatorenal fossa (1) to the right subphrenic space (3) or inferiorly along the right paracolic gutter (4) deep into the pelvis (5). Fluid also may flow from the right inframesocolic space (7) and pass over the small bowel mesentery to the left inframesocolic space (6), and may enter the pelvis (5). Fluid from the pelvis may communicate with the left paracolic gutter (8). However, fluid is blocked from ascending from the left paracolic gutter (8) to the left subphrenic space by the phrenicocolic ligament. The bare area of the liver prevents communication from the right subphrenic space into the left subphrenic space. (From Jeffrey RB Jr, McGahan JP. Gastrointestinal tract and peritoneal cavity. In: McGahan JP, Goldberg B, eds. *Diagnostic Ultrasound: A Logical Approach*. Philadelphia: Lippincott-Raven Publishers, 1998:540 with permission.)

portion of the peritoneal cavity and is often the site for initial localization of fluid collections, hemorrhage, or abscesses (Figs. 5–12 to 5–14).

It is important to understand the compartmental anatomy of the abdomen when trying to understand where fluid collections, abscesses, or hematomas are localized.[11,12]

The peritoneal compartments are subdivided based on their relationship to the transverse mesocolon (Fig. 5–11). Four intraperitoneal spaces are located within the supramesocolic portion of the abdomen. The supramesocolic spaces lie between the diaphragm and the transverse mesocolon and include the following: (1) the *right*

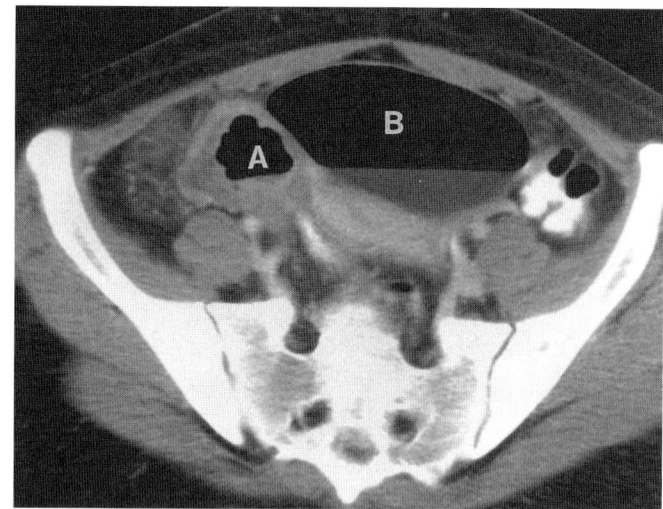

Figure 5–12 Crohn's abscess. **(A)** A contrast-enhanced computed tomogram in a 19-year-old woman with Crohn's disease who presented with right lower quadrant (RLQ) pain and fever. An RLQ abscess (A) with a gas-liquid level adjacent to the urinary bladder (B) is seen. A larger gas-liquid level is seen in the urinary bladder consistent with a fistula. Delayed images through the urinary bladder when contrast material has reached the bladder can help to distinguish fluid collections in the pelvis. **(B)** The same patient and the same examination showing one of the complications of intraperitoneal abscesses. Multiple low attenuation fluid collections in the liver represent clustered pyogenic abscesses. This shows a difficulty in achieving drainage.

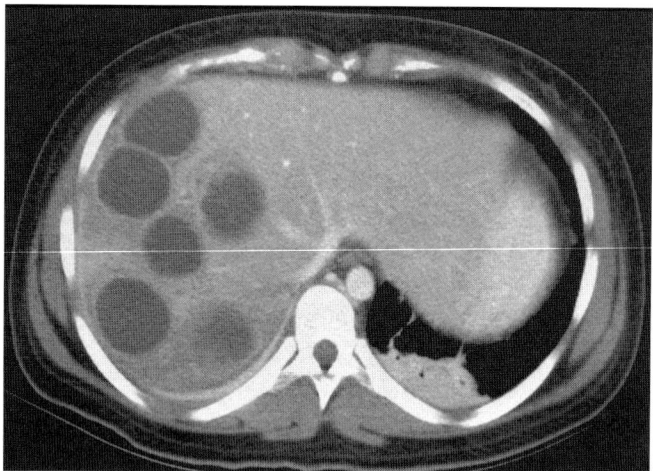

Figure 5–13 Splenic trauma. **(A)** CT examination demonstrating splenic injury (*arrows*) in this patient after a motor vehicle accident. No fluid was identified around the spleen; however, **(B)** CT scanning through the pelvis demonstrated the presence of free fluid (F) within the pelvis due to the splenic laceration. This demonstrates free flow of blood from the splenic laceration through the left paracolic gutter into the pelvis.

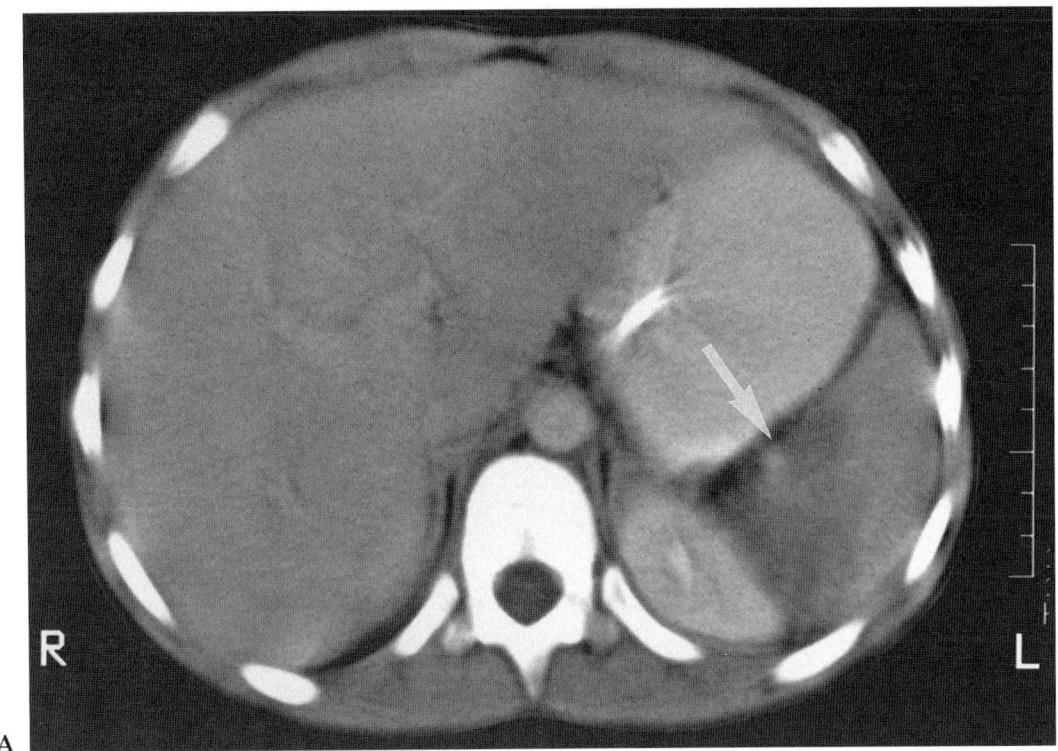

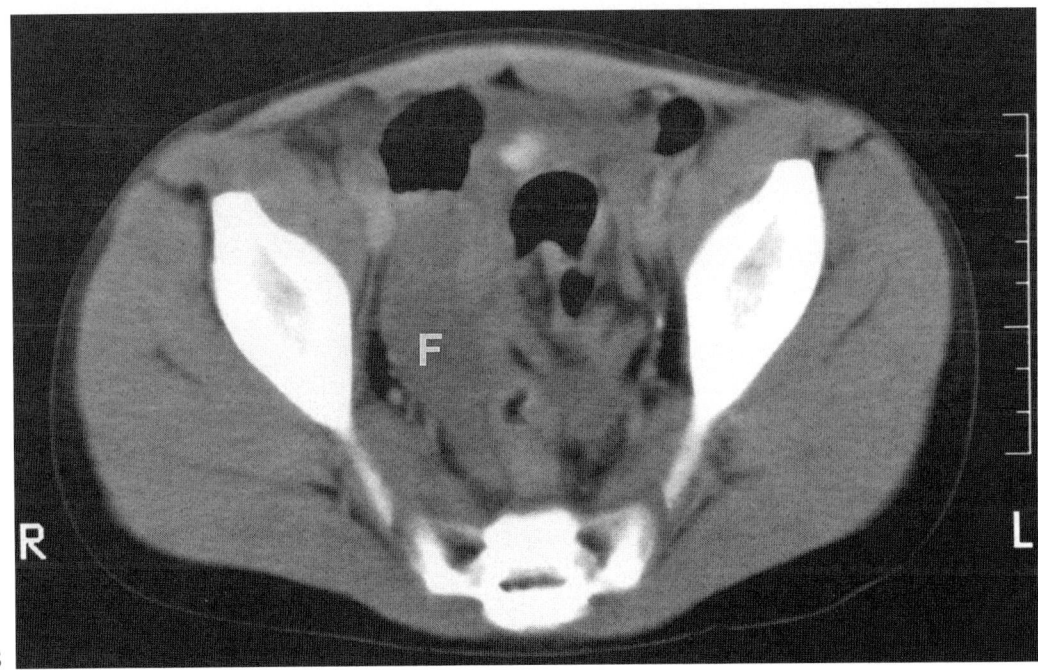

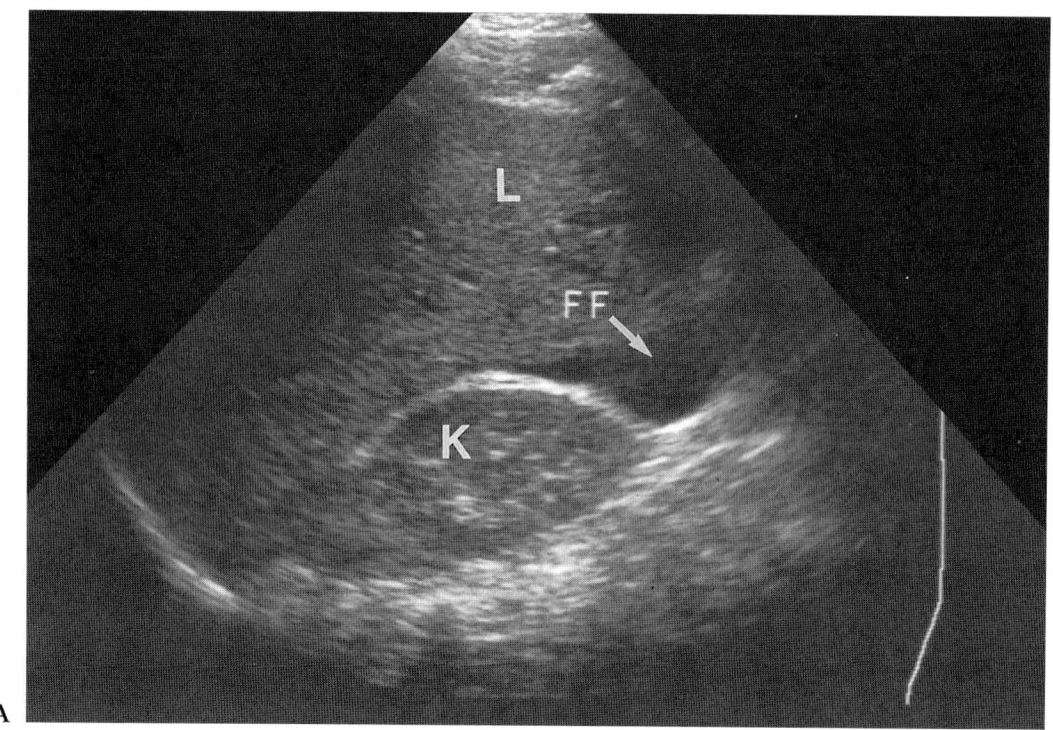

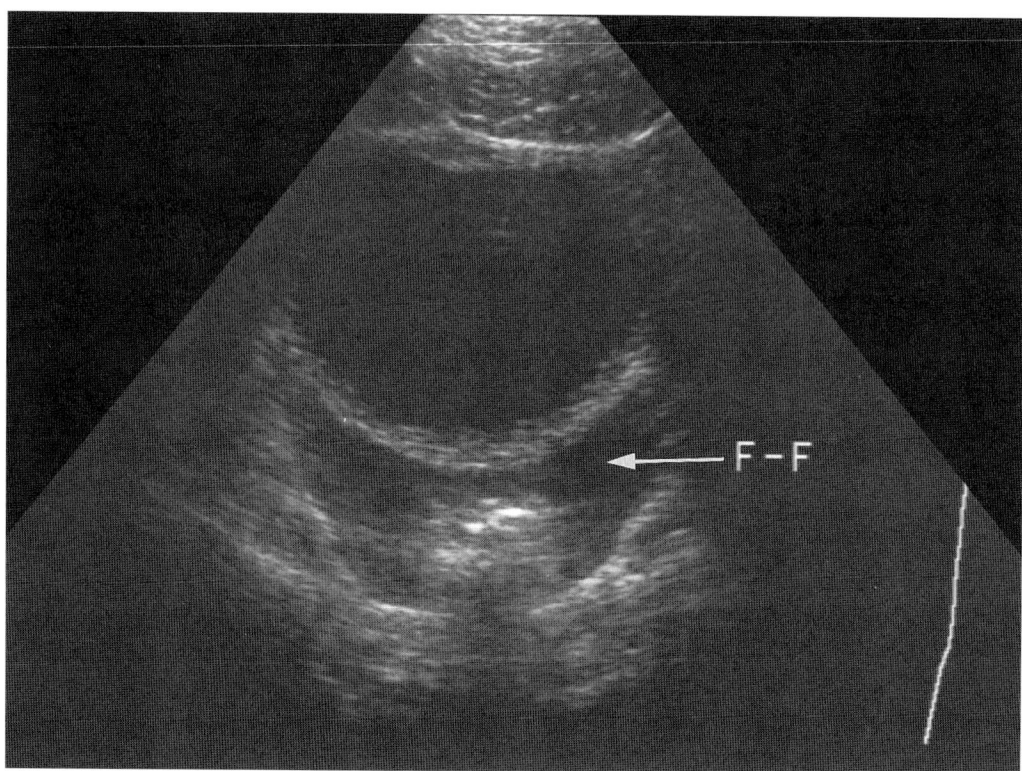

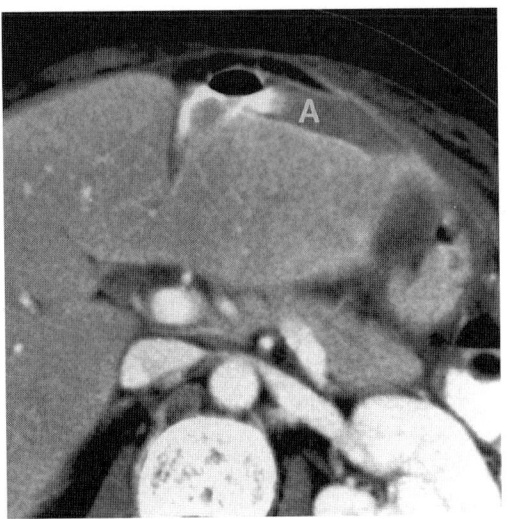

Figure 5–15 Left anterior subhepatic space. Contrast-enhanced computed tomogram in a 61-year-old man with midepigastric pain shows a rim-enhancing fluid collection in the anterior space (A). Free intraperitoneal gas and oral contrast material within the fluid collection are also seen. A perforated gastric ulcer was confirmed intraoperatively.

subhepatic space lying between the right kidney and liver, also called *Morrison's pouch* (Fig. 5–14); (2) the lesser sac (Fig. 5–10); and (3) the *right suprahepatic space*, also identified as the right subphrenic space, and the *left subphrenic space*. Infection from any of these organs can spread to the retroperitoneal spaces. Fluid can accumulate in the left subhepatic space either anterior or posterior to the liver (Figs. 5–15 and 5–16). The infracolic portion of the peritoneal cavity is divided by the small bowel mesentery into the *right inframesocolic space* (7) and the larger *left inframesocolic space* (6). These spaces may communicate with the most dependent portion of the peritoneal cavity, the pelvic cul-de-sac (5). The intraperitoneal pelvic spaces communicate with the right paracolic gutter (4) or the left paracolic gutter (8). Thus, abscesses arising in these spaces often localize in the pelvis (Figs. 5–13 and 5–14). This should be taken into account, depending on patient presentation (i.e., pelvic pain), when considering the intraperitoneal sites of origin. Alternatively, when scanning patients with paracolic gutter disease, the pelvis should be imaged routinely.[12]

Some peritoneal spaces are contiguous. Other spaces do not communicate freely due to their separation by ligamentous attachments. As an example, fluid from the subhepatic space or Morrison's pouch may communicate with the lesser sac through the foramen of Winslow. However, fluid cannot flow between the left subphrenic space and the left paracolic gutter because it is blocked by the phrenicocolic ligament. Furthermore, fluid from the subhepatic space may spread to the right subphrenic space but not the left subphrenic space because it is blocked by the bare area of the liver. An understanding of the compartmental anatomy of the abdomen is important when identifying the site of origin and where fluid may collect or abscess may develop, and in planning percutaneous therapy.

Abdominal Fluid/Abscess

Nearly half of intra-abdominal abscesses are postoperative and are located in the subphrenic area. Abscesses are located in the region of previous surgery but may extend to other sites in the abdomen. The common

Figure 5–14 Hepatic laceration. **(A)** Longitudinal ultrasonographic image of the right upper quadrant of the abdomen demonstrates evidence of free fluid (FF) in the hepatorenal fossa from recent hepatic trauma. (L) liver; (K) kidney. **(B)** Transverse scan through the patient's pelvis demonstrates free fluid posterior to the bladder. This demonstrates communication from the hepatorenal fossa through the right pericolic gutter into the pelvis.

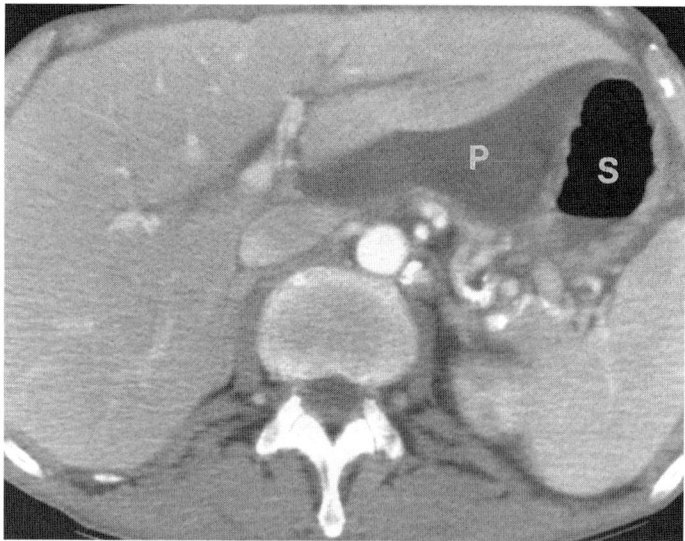

Figure 5–16 Left posterior subhepatic space. Contrast-enhanced computed tomogram in a 69-year-old man following resection of a rectal neoplasm. Patient presented with fever and an elevated white blood cell count. Shown is a large fluid collection in the left posterior subhepatic space (P). The fluid collection was successfully drained percutaneously under computed tomographic guidance. (S) stomach.

locations of the intraperitoneal abscesses are in the right and left subphrenic space, subhepatic space, hepatorenal fossa, lesser sac, left and right paracolic gutter, and pelvis[12] (Fig. 5–17). Although the subphrenic region is a common location for abscesses, the pelvis must always be carefully evaluated. This is especially true in patients who have a lower abdominal abscess that may communicate with the pelvis. Abscesses often localize to the most dependent portion of the abdomen (i.e., the pelvic cul-de-sac). For instance, in a patient with appendicitis, an abscess may be localized in the deep pelvis or even in the retroperitoneum. Another common location of abscesses includes the lesser sac. The lesser sac communicates directly with the rest of the intraperitoneal cavity through the foramen of Winslow. Commonly, lesser sac abscesses are caused by perforation of the stomach or extension of an abscess from the pancreas. Pancreatic fluid may dissect into the lesser sac and become loculated.

CT and Ultrasonographic Appearance (Abscesses)

Some of the complex anatomical relationships of the peritoneal cavity are best understood with CT.[13–15] For example, fluid collections or abscesses localized in the lesser sac, the retroperitoneal cavity, or intraperitoneal loops of bowel are well evaluated with CT. Ultrasonography is more useful in evaluating localized fluid collections, and CT gives a more global assessment. Ultrasonography is often chosen as the method to guide needle placement in performance of aspiration or drainage because of the real-time control.

Computed tomography is an excellent

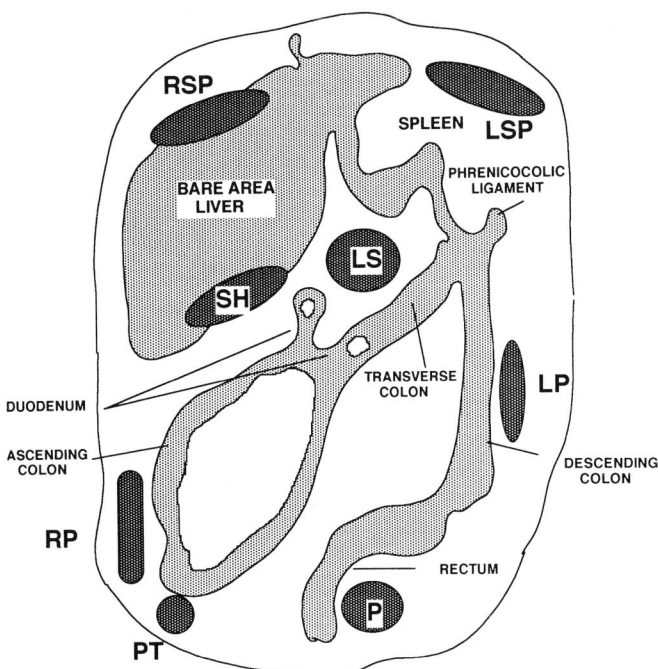

Figure 5–17 Common locations for abscess formation. Abscesses are commonly localized to the right subphrenic space (RSP) and the left subphrenic space (LSP). Abscesses also may occur in the subhepatic space (SH) (hepatorenal fossa) or the lesser sac (LS). Intra-abdominal abscesses commonly spread to the most dependent portion of the abdomen. Thus, pelvic abscesses (P) are common and should not be overlooked in patients with upper abdominal disease. Other locations for intra-abdominal abscesses include the right paracolic gutter (RP), the left paracolic gutter (LP), and the periterminal ileum (PT). (From Jeffrey RB Jr, McGahan JP. Gastrointestinal tract and peritoneal cavity. In: McGahan JP, Goldberg B, eds. *Diagnostic Ultrasound. A Logical Approach*. Philadelphia: Lippincott-Raven Publishers, 1998:550 (with permission).

noninvasive method of detecting intraperitoneal abscesses.[16] The advantages of CT are that it is noninvasive, it can easily distinguish loops of contrast-filled bowel from abscesses, and it can be helpful in identifying ectopic gas or fluid collections occurring with abscesses. CT may also be used to guide needle aspiration or drainage of abscesses.[11,17]

The CT appearance of intra-abdominal, retroperitoneal, or pelvic abscess is usually quite characteristic. These are fairly well demarcated low-attenuation masses with

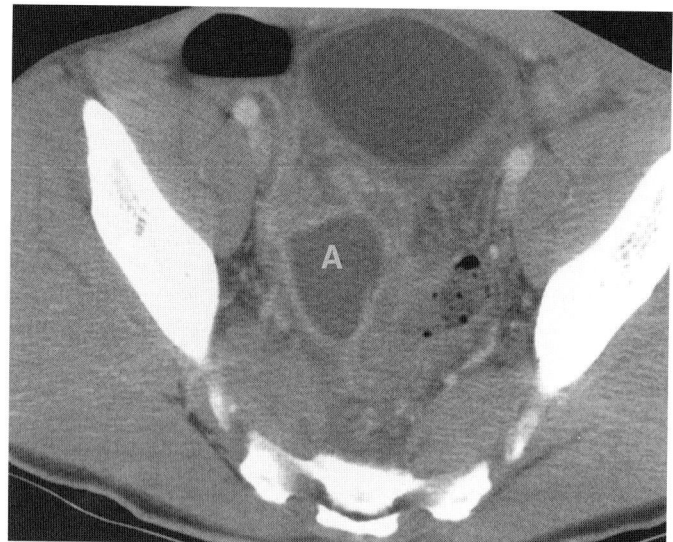

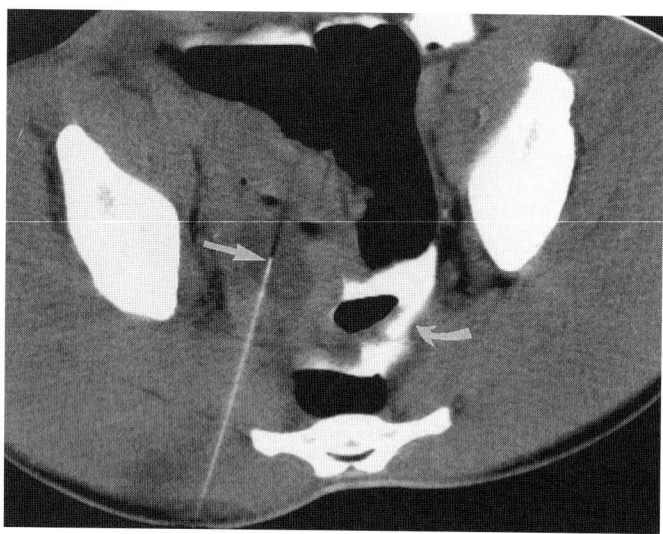

Figure 5–18 Value of rectal contrast in gastrointestinal intervention. **(A)** An enhancing fluid collection (A) in the pelvis in a 33-year-old man with a ruptured appendix. **(B)** The patient prone with added rectal contrast (*curved arrows*) to aid in differentiating fluid-filled sigmoid from the abscess prior to drainage placement. Note needle tip (*arrow*).

ill-defined or regular margins (Figs. 5–18 and 5–19). Often the periphery of the abscess cavity is very well defined and may show contrast enhancement. Alternatively, the central area of the abscess is of low attenuation (usually about that of water or slightly higher). The CT attenuation may be due to the presence of proteinaceous materials, debris, or previous hemorrhage. Gas is often present in the intra-abdominal abscess

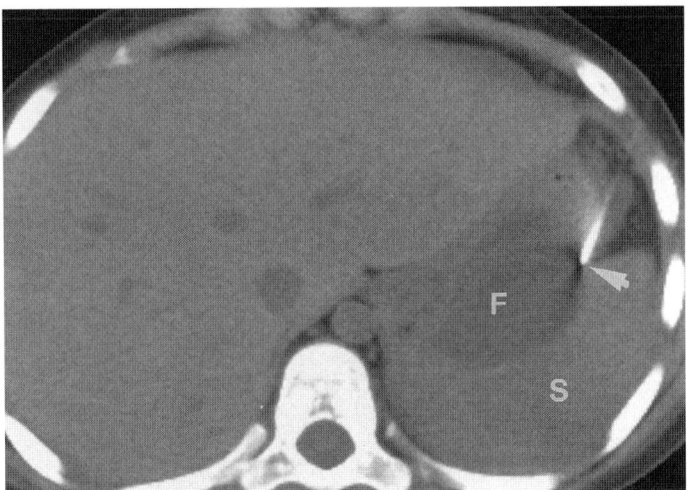

Figure 5–19 An abscess of the splenic hilum. Contrast-enhanced computed tomogram in a 9-year-old girl with a perforated appendix with persistent fever and elevated white blood cell count after appendectomy shows a low attenuation fluid collection in the splenic hilum (F). Shown is the drainage needle (*arrow*) passing between the stomach and the spleen (S). Approximately 60 cm^3 of purulent material was removed. A drain was not left in place for fear of damaging the highly vascular bed in this region. The patient subsequently improved on antibiotic therapy.

(Fig. 5–12). The gas is usually stippled throughout or may be associated with an air-fluid level. Gas may be secondary either to fistulous communication with bowel or to gas-forming organisms. On occasion, septations are visualized within the abscess with CT, but these are often better seen with sonography.[18–21]

Abscesses also may be readily detectable by ultrasonography.[22,23] Ultrasonography is most helpful in situations where the patient has a focal area of tenderness. For instance, in the postoperative patient who develops pain after a cholecystectomy, ultrasonography may be helpful in identifying an abnormal fluid collection. Ultrasonography may be used to guide aspiration and to determine if the fluid is bilious, serous, or infected.[24]

The sonographic appearance of abscesses is variable.[23] These usually are hypoechoic to anechoic and often have septations and mass effect. Abscesses usually have irregular borders. However, there are several pitfalls if ultrasonography is used as the primary method of diagnosing abdominal abscesses. Gas-filled abscesses may be densely echogenic with acoustic shadowing.[22] Reverberation artifact may occur with an air-fluid level within the abscess. These may be difficult to visualize and should not be overlooked. Also, some abdominal abscesses may appear to be solid and may be misinterpreted as an intra-abdominal mass.[23] In general, CT is used as the method of choice in diagnosing, localizing, and determining the extent of an intra-abdominal pelvic abscess. Ultrasonography is used when there is a focal area of tenderness or suspected abnormality. Both CT and ultrasonography may be utilized to guide abscess drainage. Ultrasonography is often chosen because it affords real-time control and because its portability is an advantage for fluid collection drainage in the intensive care unit.[25,26]

Other Intraperitoneal Fluid Collections

Other intraperitoneal fluid collections include ascites, bilomas, hemorrhage, lymphoceles, pancreatic pseudocysts, and urinomas.[27]

Prior to aspiration or drainage, the interventionalist may not be able to determine the exact type of fluid collection to be done. There is considerable overlap in the appearance of these fluid collections. Ascitic fluid may flow freely throughout the abdomen or may be loculated because of concurrent adhesions. Bile may be present in the peritoneal cavity following a bile leak from a recent cholecystectomy or biliary or liver surgery.[28] Urine may be present in the abdomen, especially in renal transplant patients. Other fluid collections secondary to disrupted lymphatics from previous surgery may localize as a lymphocele. Hematomas may occur in the peritoneal cavity in the postoperative patient. Finally, any fluid collection may become infected and present as an abdominal abscess. Knowledge of compartmental anatomy is important in guiding diagnostic or therapeutic aspiration or drainage of these fluid collections. Although patient history and imaging results are important in differentiating fluid collections, at times only needle aspiration can provide a definitive diagnosis and thereby direct therapy.

Summary

Knowledge of compartmental anatomy is necessary for an understanding of the origin of an abscess and for controlling the spread of infection. Proper patient assesment with CT and ultrasonography is a critical aspect of the planning of percutaneous needle aspiration or drainage. Understanding compartmental anatomy will enable the clinician to plan appropriate therapy, ensure success, and avoid potential pitfalls in the performance of percutaneous interventional procedures in the abdomen or pelvis.

References

1. Alexander ES, Proto AV, Clark RA. CT differentiation of subphrenic abscess and pleural effusion. *Am J Roentgenol* 1983; 140:47–51.
2. Gore RM. Ascites and peritoneal fluid collections. In: Gore RM, Levine MS, Laufer I, eds. *Textbook of Gastrointestinal Radiology*. Philadelphia: WB Saunders; 1994:2352.
3. Griffin DH, Gross BH, McCracken S, et al. Observation on CT differentiation of pleural and peritoneal fluid. *J Comput Assist Tomogr* 1984;8:24–28.
4. Halvorsen RA, Fedyshin PJ, Korobkin M, et al. Ascites or pleural effusion? CT differentiation: four useful criteria. *Radiographics* 1986:6:135–149.
5. Meyers MA, Whalen JP, Peelle K, et al. Radiologic features of extraperitoneal effusions: an anatomic approach. *Radiology* 1972;104:249–257.
6. Meyers MA. *Dynamic Radiology of the Abdomen: Normal and Pathologic Anatomy*. 3rd ed. New York: Springer-Verlag, 1988:179–278.
7. Hopper KD, Sherman JL, Williams MD, et al. The variable anteroposterior position of the retroperitoneal colon to the kidneys. *Invest Radiol* 1987;22:298–302.
8. Hopper KD, Sherman JL, Leuthke JM, et al. The retrorenal colon in the supine and prone patient. *Radiology* 1987;162:443–446.
9. Meyers MA. Metastatic seeding along small bowel mesentery. Roentgen features. *Am J Roentgenol* 1975;123:67–73.
10. Meyers MA. The spread and location of acute intraperitoneal effusions. *Radiology* 1970;95:547–554.
11. Jeffrey RB. Abdominal abscesses: the role of CT and sonography. In: McGahan JP, ed. *Interventional Ultrasound*. Baltimore: Williams & Wilkins; 1990:129–144.

12. Jeffrey RB, McGahan JP. Gastrointestinal tract of peritoneal cavity. In: McGahan JP, Goldberg B, eds. *Diagnostic Ultrasound: A Logical Approach*. Philadelphia: JB Lippincott; 1998:511–560.
13. Federle MP, Crass RA, Jeffrey RB, Trunkey DD. Computed tomography in blunt abdominal trauma. *Arch Surg* 1982;117:645–650.
14. Federle MP, Jeffrey RB Jr. Hemoperitoneum studied by computed tomography. *Radiology* 1983;148:187–192.
15. Siskind BN, Malat J, Hammers L, et al. CT features of hemorrhagic malignant liver tumors. *J Comput Assist Tomogr* 1987;11:766–770.
16. Callen PW. Computed tomographic evaluation of abdominal and pelvic abscesses. *Radiology* 1979;131:171–175.
17. Jeffrey RB Jr, Federle MP, Tolentino CS. Periapendiceal inflammatory masses: CT-directed management and clinical outcome in 70 patients. *Radiology* 1988;167:13–16.
18. Gerzof SH, Johnson WC. Radiological aspects of diagnosis and treatment of abscesses. *Surg Clin North Am* 1984;64:53–66.
19. Koehler PR, Moss AA. Diagnosis of intraabdominal and pelvic abscesses by computerized tomography. *JAMA* 1980;244:49–52.
20. Mueller PR, Simeone JF. Intraabdominal abscesses: diagnosis by sonography and computed tomography. *Radiol Clin North Am* 1983;21:425–444.
21. Stafford SA, Mueller PR. Imaging abdominal abscess with ultrasound and CT. *Diagn Imaging* 1985;7:60–69.
22. Kressel HY, Filly RA. Ultrasonographic appearance of gas-containing abscesses in the abdomen. *Am J Roentgensl* 1978;130:71–73.
23. Subramanyam BR, Balthazar EJ, Raghavendra BN, Horii SC, Hilton S, Naidich DP. Ultrasound analysis of solid-appearing abscesses. *Radiology* 1983;146:487–491.
24. McGahan JP. Interventional abdominal ultrasound. In: Mittelstaedt CA, ed. *General Ultrasound*. New York: Churchill Livingstone; 1992:1189–1204.
25. McGahan JP. Aspiration and drainage procedure in the intensive care unit: percutaneous sonographic guidance. *Radiology* 1985;154:531–532.
26. McGahan JP, Anderson MW, Walter JP. Portable real-time sonographic and needle guidance systems for aspiration and drainage. *Am J Roentgenol* 1986;147:1241–1246.
27. Norwood SH, Civetta JM. Abdominal CT scanning in critically ill surgical patients. *Ann Surg* 1085;202:166–175.
28. McGahan JP, Stein M. Complications of laparoscopic cholecystectomy: imaging and intervention. *Am J Roentgenol* 1995;165:1089–1097.

Index

Page numbers in *italics* refer to tables or art.

Abscess and fluid collection, 96–114. *See also* Fluid collection and abscess
Acid suppression therapy in upper GI bleeding, 3–4, 19–20
α2-Adrenergic agonists in prevention of portal hypertensive bleeding, 3
β-Adrenergic blockers in prevention of portal hypertensive bleeding, 3
Amyotrophic lateral sclerosis, intestinal gas lock in, *82*, 83
Angiodysplasia, lower GI bleeding in, 22, *22*, *23*
  and embolization therapy, *15*
Angiography
  in lower GI bleeding, 24
  in upper GI bleeding, 11–16
    and embolization therapy, 14–16
    and vasopressin therapy, 14
Antibiotic therapy
  colonic irrigation technique, 78–79
  in *Helicobacter pylori* infections, 4, 19
Anti-inflammatory agents, gastrointestinal bleeding from, 1, 2
  acid suppression therapy in, 3
Aortic rupture, *103*
Appendix rupture, *100*, *101*, *112*
Argon plasma coagulation in upper GI bleeding, 10
Ascites, 114
  colostomy in, percutaneous, 84
  gastrostomy in, percutaneous, 53
  transjugular intrahepatic portosystemic shunting in, 17
Aspiration problems
  gastrojejunostomy in, 52, 60, *61*
  jejunostomy in, percutaneous, 67

Band ligation in upper GI hemorrhage, 11, *11*
Bard Button, 63, *66*
Bare area of liver, *97*, *98*
Billroth I procedure in peptic ulcer disease and upper GI bleeding, 21
Biloma, 114
Bipolar thermal coagulation in upper GI bleeding, 9
Bleeding, gastrointestinal, 1–24
  from lower tract, 21–24
    angiography in, 24
    colonoscopy in, 22, *22*–23, *23*, 24
    embolization therapy in, *15*, 24
    surgical techniques in, 24
    vasopressin therapy in, *14*
  mortality in, 1, 2
  from upper tract, 2–21
    acid suppression therapy in, 3–4, 19–20
    angiography in, 11–16
    band ligation in, 11, *11*
    clip placement in, 10
    diagnostic endoscopy in, 4–5, *5*, *6*
    embolization therapy in, 14–16
    Helicobacter pylori eradication in, 4, 19
    injection therapy in, endoscopic, 5–9
    medical resuscitation in, 2
    nuclear scintigraphy in, 11, *12*
    pharmacologic control of, 2–4
    prediction of rebleeding rates in, 5
    surgical management of, 19–21
    tattooing in, endoscopic, 11
    thermal coagulation techniques in, *9*, 9–10

INDEX

Bleeding, gastrointestinal (*Continued*)
    transjugular intrahepatic portosystemic shunts in, 16–19
    vasopressin therapy in, 14
Boerhaave's syndrome, esophageal stenting in, 42
n-Butyl-2-cyanoacrylate glue in esophageal leaks and fistula, 43, 44, 45

Calopinto needle in TIPSS, 17–19, *18*
Carcinoma. *See* Tumors
Carcinomatosis, gastric, percutaneous gastrostomy in, 53
Cardiovascular changes in TIPSS, 16
Carey-Alzate-Coons gastrojejunostomy catheters, 63, *65*
Cecostomy
    antibiotic instillation in, 78–79
    in children, 90
    in constipation and fecal incontinence, 78
    detorsion of cecal volvulus in, 80
Cecum
    decompression of, percutaneous colostomy in, 77–78
    volvulus of, 77, 80, 90
        perforation in, 80, *81*
Celiac artery angiography in upper GI bleeding, 12, 13, *13*
Cerebrovascular disorders, percutaneous gastrostomy in, 52, *58–59*
Children, cecostomy in, 90
Cirrhosis, upper GI bleeding in, 2, 3
Clip placement, endoscopic, in upper GI bleeding, 10
Clonidine, in prevention of portal hypertensive bleeding, 3
Coagulation disorders
    colostomy in, percutaneous, 84
    gastrostomy in, 53, 69
Colitis
    ischemic, lower GI bleeding in, 22, 23
    pseudomembranous, colonic irrigation with antibiotics in, 78–79
    radiation-induced, lower GI bleeding in, 22, 24
Colon
    accidental puncture in percutaneous nephrostomy, 84
    irrigation of
        with antibiotics in colitis therapy, 78–79
        in constipation and fecal incontinence, 78, *79*, *80*
    obstruction and pseudo-obstruction of, 77–78, 91
        access site and tube placement in, 84–86, 91
        drainage enterostomy in, 80
        in gas locks, 83–84
        recommended colostomy technique in, 91–92
    stenting of, 46–47
        indications for, 46, 80
        insertion technique in, 46–47
        results of, 47
Colonoscopy in lower GI bleeding, *22*, 22–23, *23*, *24*
Colostomy, percutaneous, 77–93
    in cecal decompression, 77–78, 93
    in cecal volvulus, 80, 90
    contraindications to, 84
    for drainage, 84, 91–92
        distal and proximal arrangement in, *87*, *88*
        indications for, 80
        leakage affecting, 86
    entry site in, 84–86, 91
    equipment options in, 90–91, 92, *92*
    fixation devices in, 87–90, *89*, 92
    indications for, 77–84
    in intestinal gas locks, *82*, *83*, 83–84
    for irrigation
        in colitis and antibiotic therapy, 78–79
        in constipation and fecal incontinence, 78, *79*, *80*
    leakage problems in, 86, *86*
    in Ogilvie's syndrome, 77–78, 90, 93
    postprocedure management in, 93
    retroperitoneal and transperitoneal approaches in, 90
    sedation and anesthesia in, 91
    technical considerations in, 84–91
Computed tomography
    in fluid collection and abscess, 110–14
        in aortic rupture, *103*
        bare area of liver in, *97*
        in Crohn's disease, *106*
        in diverticulitis, *97*, *101*
        in duodenal perforation, *102*

118

in pancreatic abscess, *99, 104*
in pancreatitis, *99*
in splenic laceration, *107*
in subhepatic space, *109, 110*
in jejunostomy after gastrectomy, 56
in upper GI bleeding, 13
Constipation, colonic irrigation in, 78, *79*
Crohn's disease
    intraperitoneal abscess in, *106*
    lower GI bleeding in, 22
Cystic fibrosis, colonic irrigation in, 78, *80*

Decompression of bowel
    colostomy in, percutaneous, 77–78
    gastrostomy in, 51, 52
Dieulafoy's vascular malformation, 4
    endoscopic tattooing in, 11
    thermal coagulation techniques in, 9, *9*
Displaced crus sign, 98
Diverticula
    fluid collection and abscess in, *96, 97, 101*
    lower GI bleeding in, 22, *23*
Drainage procedures
    colostomy in, percutaneous, 84, 91–92
        distal and proximal arrangement in, *87, 88*
        indications for, 80
        leakage affecting, 86
    peritoneal and retroperitoneal anatomy in, 96–114
Duodenostomy, percutaneous translumbar, 67
Duodenum
    in anterior pararenal space, 102, *102*
    bleeding from, in peptic ulcer disease, 3, 19–21. *See also* Peptic ulcer disease and upper GI bleeding
    retroperitoneal perforation of, *102*
    stenting of, 45–46
Dysphagia
    esophageal stenting in, 35–45
        in benign disease, 41–42
        in malignant disease, *39*, 39–40, *40*, 41
    gastrostomy in, 51, 52

Elderly, gastrointestinal bleeding in, 1, 2
    surgery in, 20, 21

Embolization therapy
    in lower GI bleeding, *15*, 24
    in upper GI bleeding, 14–16
Emergency surgery in upper GI bleeding, 20, 21
Encephalopathy, hepatic, in TIPSS, 16
Endoscopy
    gastrostomy in, percutaneous. *See* Gastrostomy, percutaneous endoscopic
    in upper GI bleeding
        band ligation in, 11, *11*
        clip placement in, 10
        in diagnosis, 4–5, *5, 6*
        injection therapy in, 5–9
        tattooing of lesions in, 11
Enteral nutrition
    compared to parenteral nutrition, 52
    indications for gastrostomy in, 51–52
Enteroscopy, diagnostic, in upper GI bleeding, 4–5
Enterostomy
    for drainage in intestinal obstruction, 80
    fixation devices in, 87, 89
    in intestinal ischemia, 85
    leakage problems in, 86, 89
Epinephrine, in endoscopic injection therapy for upper GI bleeding, 7–9
Esophagitis, upper GI bleeding and acid suppression therapy in, 3
Esophagus
    carcinoma of, stenting in. *See* Tumors, esophageal stenting in
    hemorrhage from
        in esophagitis or esophageal ulcers, 3
        in varices. *See* Variceal hemorrhage
    stenting of, 35–45
        in benign strictures, 35, 41–42, *42*
        complications of, 37, 39–40, *40, 42, 42*
        insertion technique in, 37, *38*
        in leaks and fistula of esophagus, 35, 42–45
        in malignant disease. *See* Tumors, esophageal stenting in
        types of stents in, 35–37
Ethanol, in endoscopic injection therapy for upper GI bleeding, 7–9

Feces
  evacuation of, 91
    colonic irrigation in, 78, *79, 80*
    drainage enterostomy in, 80
    stenting in, 80
  incontinence of, colonic irrigation in, 78
Fistula, tracheoesophageal
  after esophageal stenting, 39, *40*
  esophageal stenting in, 35, 42, *44*
Fixation devices in percutaneous colostomy, 87–90, *89*, 92
Fluid collection and abscess, 96–114
  computed tomography in. *See* Computed tomography, in fluid collection and abscess
  in peritoneum, 104–14
  in retroperitoneum, 99–103
  supradiaphragmatic and subdiaphragmatic, 96–99, *98*
  signs of, *97*, 98
  ultrasonography in, *98*, 99, 110, 113–14
  in hepatic laceration, *108*
Foramen of Winslow, *105*, 109, 110

Gas locks, intestinal, percutaneous colostomy in, *82, 83*, 83–84
Gastrectomy
  percutaneous gastrostomy with balloon technique in, 65–66
  percutaneous jejunostomy in, 53, *56–57*
Gastric outlet obstruction
  gastroenterostomy in, 45
  jejunostomy in, percutaneous, 67
  stenting in, 45–46, *46*
Gastritis, stress, in ventilatory support, 4
Gastroduodenal artery
  angiography in upper GI bleeding, 13, *13*
  embolization in upper GI bleeding, 15
Gastroenterostomy
  in gastric outlet obstruction, 45
  percutaneous, 51–72
Gastroesophageal reflux
  in esophageal stenting, 37
  in gastrostomy, 52
Gastrointestinal bleeding. *See* Bleeding, gastrointestinal

Gastrojejunostomy
  after percutaneous endoscopic gastrostomy, 60–61, *62*
  indications for, 52, 60
  infracolic approach, 66–67
  technique and materials in, 60–61, *61, 62–63*
Gastropathy in portal hypertension, 3, 4
Gastropexy in percutaneous gastrostomy, 57–59, 69
Gastrostomy
  percutaneous, 51–72
    in cerebrovascular disorders, 52, *58–59*
    contraindications to, 52–53
    fixation devices in, 87–89, *89*
    gastropexy in, 57–59, 69
    hydrophilic coating of catheters in, 62–63, *64*
    indications for, 51–52
    migration of tube in, 70, *71, 72*
    in Parkinson's disease, 69, *70*
    puncture site in, 55
    repositioning of catheter in, 70, *71*
    results and complications in, 68–71
    technique and materials in, 53–67
  percutaneous endoscopic, 51, 53
    aspiration problems in, 60
    conversion to gastrojejunostomy, 60–61, *62*
    migration of tube in, *71*
    results and complications in, 60, 68–69, 70
    technical variations in, 68
  surgical, 51, 53
    results and complications in, 68, 69
Gelfoam embolization
  in lower GI bleeding, 24
  in upper GI bleeding, 14–15
Gianturco stent, esophageal, 35, 37
  in benign stricture, *42*

Heater probe devices
  in lower GI bleeding, 22
  in upper GI bleeding, 9–10
Helicobacter pylori infections, 1
  upper GI bleeding in, 4, 19
Hemangioma, cavernous, recurrent GI bleeding in, *12*

120

Hemorrhage, gastrointestinal. *See* Bleeding, gastrointestinal
Hemorrhoids, lower GI bleeding in, 22
Hepatic artery embolization in upper GI bleeding, 16
Hepatic space, right (Morrison's pouch), 105, *105,* 109
Hepatorenal fossa (subhepatic space), *105,* 110, *111*
  left anterior, *109*
  left posterior, *110*
Historical aspects of gastrostomy, 51
HIV infection
  gastrojejunostomy in, *61*
  rectal ulcers in, *14*
Hypertension, portal, upper GI bleeding in, 3
  sclerotherapy in, 5–7
  transjugular intrahepatic portosystemic shunts in, 16–19

Incontinence, fecal, colonic irrigation in, 78
Inframesocolic space, *105,* 109
Injection therapy, endoscopic, in upper GI bleeding, 5–9
  in varices, 5–7, *7, 8*
  in visible vessels and mucosal tears, 7–9
Interface sign, 98
Irrigation of colon
  with antibiotics in colitis therapy, 78–79
  in constipation and fecal incontinence, 78, *79, 80*
Ischemia, intestinal
  colitis and lower GI bleeding in, 22, *23*
  obstruction and percutaneous drainage in, 85, *86*

Jejunostomy
  for early postoperative nutrition, 52
  percutaneous, 51–72
    fixation devices in, 87, *89*
    in gastrectomy, 53, *56–57*
    in pulmonary disease and cardiomyopathy, 54
    technique in, *54, 56–57,* 67
  percutaneous endoscopic, 67
Jejunum, advancement of feeding catheter to, 52, *60–61*

Kidneys
  and anatomy of retroperitoneum, 101–3
    anterior pararenal, 102–3
    perirenal, 101–2
    posterior pararenal, 103
  in perinephric abscess, *100,* 101
  in transjugular intrahepatic portosystemic shunting, 16, 17

Laceration
  of liver, *108*
  of spleen, *107*
Laparoscopy, in peptic ulcer disease and upper GI bleeding, 21
Laser therapy
  in esophageal carcinoma, compared to stenting, 41
  in lower GI bleeding, 22
  in upper GI bleeding, 10
Liver
  bare area of, *97,* 98
  in transjugular intrahepatic portosystemic shunting, 16–19
Lower GI bleeding, 21–24
Lymphocele, 114

Mallory–Weiss tears, 4
  embolization therapy in, 15
Meningomyelocele, colonic irrigation for constipation in, 79
Mesenteric artery angiography
  inferior
    in lower GI bleeding, 24
    in upper GI bleeding, 13, *14*
  superior
    in lower GI bleeding, 24
    in upper GI bleeding, 12, *12,* 13
MIC–Key device, 63, *66*
Monopolar thermal coagulation techniques
  in lower GI bleeding, 22
  in upper GI bleeding, 9
Morrison's pouch (right hepatic space), 105, *105,* 109
Multipolar thermal coagulation techniques
  in lower GI bleeding, 22
  in upper GI bleeding, 9

Nadolol, in prevention of portal hypertensive bleeding, 3
Nasogastric intubation
 for nutritional support, 52
 prior to percutaneous gastrostomy, 53, 55
 in upper GI bleeding, 2
Nd:YAG laser therapy in upper GI bleeding, 10
Nephrostomy, percutaneous, accidental puncture of colon in, 84
Nitrates, in prevention of portal hypertensive bleeding, 3
Nitroglycerin with vasopressin in GI bleeding, 2
Nuclear scintigraphy in upper GI bleeding, 11, *12*
Nutritional support
 gastrojejunostomy in, 52, 60, *61*
 gastrostomy in, 51
  in cerebrovascular accident, *58–59*
  first feeding in, 56–57
  indications for, 51–52
  in Parkinson's disease, 69, *70*
 jejunostomy in, *54*, 56–57
 nasogastric feeding tubes in, 52

Octreotide in GI bleeding, 2–3
Ogilvie's syndrome
 in colonic gas locks, 83–84
 percutaneous colostomy in, 77–78, 90, 93

Pancreas
 abscess of, *99, 104*, 110
 pseudocyst of, 99, *99*, 114
Pancreaticoduodenal arcade embolization in upper GI bleeding, 15
Paracolic gutters, *105*, 109
Pararenal space, anatomy of, 102–3
Parenteral nutrition, compared to enteral nutrition, 52
Parkinson's disease, gastrostomy for nutritional support in, 69, *70*
Peptic ulcer disease and upper GI bleeding
 acid suppression therapy in, 3, 19–20
 diagnostic endoscopy in, 4, *5, 6*

Helicobacter pylori eradication in, 4, 19
 injection therapy in, endoscopic, 7
 surgical management of, 19–21
 thermal coagulation techniques in, 9, 10
Percutaneous approach
 in colostomy, 77–93
 in gastrostomy, gastroenterostomy, and jejunostomy, 51–72
 in nephrostomy, accidental puncture of colon in, 84
 peritoneal and retroperitoneal anatomy in, 96–114
Perirenal or perinephric space
 anatomy of, *101*, 101–2
 in rupture of retrocecal appendix, *100*, 101
 septa of, *99*, 102
Peritoneal sac
 greater, 104
 lesser, 104, *105*, 109, 110
Peritoneum
 fluid collection and abscess in, 104–14
  computed tomography in, 110–14
  in Crohn's disease, *106*
  spread of fluid in, *105*
  ultrasonography in, *108*, 110, 113–14
 in percutaneous colostomy approach, 90
Portal hypertension, upper GI bleeding in, 3
 sclerotherapy in, 5–7
 transjugular intrahepatic portosystemic shunts in, 16–19
Portosystemic shunts, transjugular intrahepatic, 16–19, *18*
Propranolol, in prevention of portal hypertensive bleeding, 3
Proton pump inhibitors in upper GI bleeding, 3, 20
Pseudocyst of pancreas, 99, *99*, 114
Pseudo-obstruction, intestinal, percutaneous colostomy in, 77–78

Radiation
 colitis from, lower GI bleeding in, 22, *24*
 in esophageal carcinoma therapy, compared to stenting, 41
Radionuclide scans in upper GI bleeding, 11, *12*
Rectal ulcers in HIV infection, *14*

Rectosigmoid stenting, 46–47
Red cell scanning in upper GI bleeding, 11, *12*
Reflux, gastroesophageal
  in esophageal stenting, 37
  in gastrostomy, 52
Resuscitation measures
  in lower GI bleeding, 21–22
  in upper GI bleeding, 2
Retroperitoneum
  fluid collection and abscess in, 99–103
  in percutaneous colostomy approach, 90

Sclerosis, amyotrophic lateral, intestinal gas lock in, *82*, 83
Sclerotherapy in upper GI bleeding, 5–7, *7, 8*
  agents used in, 5
  compared to drug therapy, 3
Shock
  in lower GI bleeding, 24
  in upper GI bleeding, 2
    surgery in, 20
Shunts, transjugular intrahepatic portosystemic, 16–19, *18*
Splenic trauma, *107*
Stents, 35–47
  colonic, 46–47, 80
  esophageal, 35–45. *See also* Esophagus, stenting of
  gastric antral and duodenal, 45–46
  in transjugular intrahepatic portosystemic shunting, *18*, 19
Stomach
  bleeding from
    in peptic ulcer disease, 3, 19–21. *See also* Peptic ulcer disease and upper GI bleeding
    in portal hypertensive gastropathy, 3
    in varices, 3, 4, 7, *8*, 17. *See also* Variceal hemorrhage
  outlet obstruction of
    gastroenterostomy in, 45
    jejunostomy in, percutaneous, 67
    stenting in, 45–46, *46*
  varices of
    hemorrhage in, 3, 4, 7, *8*, 17. *See also* Variceal hemorrhage
    percutaneous gastrostomy in, 53

Stool. *See* Feces
Strecker stent, esophageal, 35, 36–37
  insertion of, 37
  in malignant disease, *36*, 39, *40*, 41
Stress gastritis in ventilatory support, 4
Subdiaphragmatic fluid collection, 96–99
Subhepatic space (hepatorenal fossa), *105*, 110, *111*
  left anterior, *109*
  left posterior, *110*
Subphrenic (suprahepatic) space, *105*, 109, 110, *111*
Supradiaphragmatic fluid collection, 96–99
Suprahepatic (subphrenic) space, *105*, 109, 110, *111*
Supramesocolic space, 105
Surgery
  in esophageal carcinoma, compared to stenting, 41
  gastrostomy in, 51, 53
    results and complications in, 68, 69
  in lower GI bleeding, 24
  in upper GI bleeding, 19–21
    in emergency care, 20, 21
    indications for, 20–21
    operative techniques in, 21

Tattooing of lesions in upper GI bleeding, 11
Thermal coagulation techniques
  in lower GI bleeding, 22
  in upper GI bleeding, *9*, 9–10
TIPSS (transjugular intrahepatic portosystemic shunts), 16–19, *18*
Tracheoesophageal fistula
  after esophageal stenting, 39, *40*
  esophageal stenting in, 35, 42, *44*
Transfusions in upper GI bleeding, 2, 20
Transjugular intrahepatic portosystemic shunts, 16–19, *18*
Trauma
  hepatic laceration in, *108*
  splenic laceration in, *107*
T-tack fixation devices, 87–90
Tumors
  colonic stenting in, 46–47
  esophageal stenting in, 35, *36*, *38*, 39–41
    compared to other techniques, 41
    complications of, 39–40, *40*

Tumors (*Continued*)
    in leaks and fistula of esophagus, 42, 43, 44
    results of, *39*, 39–40, *40*
    gastrectomy and jejunostomy in, *56–57*
    gastric antral stenting in, 45–46, *46*

Ulcers
    of rectum in HIV infection, *14*
    upper GI bleeding in
        acid suppression therapy in, 3, 19–20
        diagnostic endoscopy in, 4, 5, *5*, *6*
        Helicobacter pylori eradication in, 4, 19
        injection therapy in, endoscopic, 7
        surgical management of, 19–21
        thermal coagulation techniques in, 9, 10
Ultrasonography in fluid collection and abscess, *98*, 99, 110, 113–14
    in hepatic laceration, *108*
Upper GI bleeding, 2–21
Urinoma, 114

Vagotomy, in peptic ulcer disease and upper GI bleeding, 21

VanSonnenberg gastrostomy catheter, 63, *63*
Variceal hemorrhage, 3
    band ligation in, 11, *11*
    diagnostic endoscopy in, 4
    drug therapy in, 3
    sclerotherapy in, 5–7, *7*, *8*
    transjugular intrahepatic portosystemic shunts in, 16–19
Vasopressin therapy in GI bleeding, 2, 14, *14*
Ventilatory support, stress gastritis in, 4
Volvulus of cecum, 77, 80, 90
    perforation in, 80, *81*

Wallstents
    esophageal, 35–36
        in leaks and fistula of esophagus, 42, 43
        in malignant disease, 39–40, *40*, 41
    in gastric outlet obstruction, 45, *46*
    rectosigmoid, 47
    in transjugular intrahepatic portosystemic shunting, *18*, 19
Wilms-Oglesby gastrojejunostomy catheter, 63, *65*
Winslow foramen, *105*, 109, 110